PENGUIN BOOKS

YOUR NAME IS HUGHES HANNIBAL SHANKS

Lela Knox Shanks is an independent scholar and lecturer living in Lincoln, Nebraska. She and Hughes Hannibal Shanks were married for fifty years and have four children. Hughes died on April 10, 1998.

Steven H. Zarit is a professor of human development and assistant director of the Gerontology Center at the Pennsylvania State University. He is also coauthor of *The Hidden Victims of Alzheimer's Disease: Families Under Stress.*

Agendas for Aging

General Editor
Theo B. Sonderegger
University of Nebraska–Lincoln [emeritus]

Series Editors
Paul B. Baltes
Max Planck Institute for Human Development and Education

Paul T. Costa Jr.
National Institute on Aging and Georgetown University
    School of Medicine

Irene M. Hulicka
State University of New York College at Buffalo

Suzanne T. Ortega
University of Nebraska–Lincoln

K. Warner Schaie
Pennsylvania State University

A Caregiver's Guide to Alzheimer's

Your Name Is

Hughes Hannibal Shanks

Lela Knox Shanks

With a foreword by Steven H. Zarit

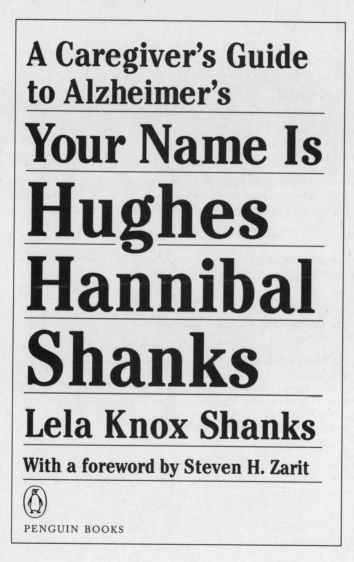

PENGUIN BOOKS

PENGUIN BOOKS
Published by the Penguin Group
Penguin Putnam Inc., 375 Hudson Street, New York, New York 10014, U.S.A.
Penguin Books Ltd, 27 Wrights Lane, London W8 5TZ, England
Penguin Books Australia Ltd, Ringwood, Victoria, Australia
Penguin Books Canada Ltd, 10 Alcorn Avenue, Toronto, Ontario, Canada M4V 3B2
Penguin Books (N.Z.) Ltd, 182–190 Wairau Road, Auckland 10, New Zealand

Penguin Books Ltd, Registered Offices: Harmondsworth, Middlesex, England

First published in the United States of America by University of Nebraska Press 1996
This edition with a new epilogue published in Penguin Books 1999

10 9 8 7 6 5 4 3

THE LIBRARY OF CONGRESS HAS CATALOGUED THE HARDCOVER AS FOLLOWS:
Shanks, Lela Knox.
Your name is Hughes Hannibal Shanks: a caregiver's guide to Alzheimer's / Lela Knox
Shanks; with a foreword by Steven H. Zarit.
p.   cm.—(Agenda for aging)
Includes bibliographical references and index.
ISBN 0-8032-4245-X (hc.)
ISBN 0 14 02.7619 X (pbk.)
1. Alzheimer's disease—Popular works.   2. Alzheimer's disease—Patients—Care.   I. Title.
II. Series.
RC523.2.S53   1996
618.97'6831—dc20   96-3691

Printed in the United States of America
Designed by A. Shahan

To Ron, Hughes's son, who died while I was writing this book;

and to Christopher, our grandson,

who came to be an active part of Hughes's life after Ron's death.

Contents

Illustrations

PHOTOS

Following page 96

TABLE

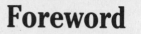

Foreword
Steven H. Zarit, Ph.D.

This remarkable book is about one family's struggle to cope with the devastating effects of Alzheimer's disease. But Lela Knox Shanks is so keen an observer and such a resolute caregiver that everyone involved in the care of older people—from physicians first making the diagnosis of Alzheimer's disease, to social workers or nurses or psychologists who work with patients and families, to aides in adult day-care or nursing home programs, and families who find themselves in similar situations—can learn something valuable from this book.

Over the past decade we have heard a great deal about the stresses of caregiving from the media as well as from scholarly research. Being the full-time caregiver for someone suffering from Alzheimer's disease or similar disorders is without question one of the most stressful and demanding roles we can take on during our lifetime. Moreover, as Lela Knox Shanks demonstrates, caregiving is usually not something we do for a short time; the demands sometimes stretch out over a period of many years. It is not surprising that caregivers frequently feel depressed, angry, or overwhelmed by their situation, or that their own health suffers in the process.

In many respects, the demands that are being placed on families by caregiving are unprecedented. Families have always cared for their elderly relatives, but the need for care has changed in substantial ways. As a result of the dramatic increases in life expectancy during the twentieth century, a greater proportion of the population is surviving to old age than ever before. Most older people are healthy and able to lead fulfilling, independent lives. But the negative side of life extension is that people are living to ages when they are at greater risk for a variety of chronic diseases such as Alzheimer's. Furthermore, the same improvements in health care that have extended our years have also contributed to an expansion of morbidity: that is, people live longer *after* developing a chronic illness. Not long ago, medical textbooks described the life expectancy of an Alzheimer's patient as two to four years. Now, patients typically survive for ten, fifteen, or even twenty years after the onset of this disease, and they need extensive care for most of that time. As a result of these changes in life expectancy, the families of elders who have severe and complex disabilities must provide more care for longer periods than ever before. Most families are not prepared for the extensive demands they will face as caregivers, nor have we as a society developed ways of effectively sharing their burden.

This book vividly captures the problems and challenges that family caregivers face: the growing awareness that something is seriously wrong with a husband or wife, a father or mother; the discovery that the usual ways of doing things and even of communicating with the patient no longer work; the frustrating process of trial and error to find out what helps; turning to others for help but sometimes not getting what is needed; and the constant challenge of adapting and changing as the situation evolves. There is also the growing sense of the loss of this person who has been loved deeply by his or her family and now is in the throes of Alzheimer's disease.

But *Your Name Is Hughes Hannibal Shanks* is more than a compilation of the stresses that families face. It is a remarkable guide to survival, of how to adapt and change as new challenges arise. Lela Knox Shanks provides us with many valuable lessons about how to cope with the particular problems of caring for someone with Alzheimer's disease. In doing so, she avoids the trap that many caregiving books fall into of saying that there is only one way to do things—her way. Instead, her lessons are about a *process* of figuring out what to do in order to get by. In the end, the most important lesson concerns learning an attitude and an approach to caregiving that makes its stresses more manageable for the long haul.

Because Lela Knox Shanks describes her experiences so eloquently, it is difficult to summarize or condense those lessons into a few pages. But I do want to point out some of the most important and powerful themes that emerge in this book.

We learn of her growing realization that her husband has a problem and that she is the one who must adjust and compensate for it. This realization is the first and, in many ways, most important transition that caregivers face. Part of the process is coming to terms with the frightening implications of a diagnosis such as Alzheimer's disease; part of it is recognizing that the care recipient can no longer regulate his or her life in some important ways. Lela Knox Shanks poignantly describes her early struggles to understand her husband's problems and what she could do about them. Like many caregivers, she was angry about changes she could not understand or explain, for taking charge means giving up hope that the problem will be cured or will just go away. But it also means starting the process of identifying the things that can be changed to make the situation better. As a man who had been caring for his wife for many years once told me, the most important thing he had learned was that he was the one who had to change.

That brings us to a second theme, that there is much that can be done to help someone with Alzheimer's disease and to make the situation a little more manageable for the caregiver. Although Alzheimer's is an irreversible, progressive disorder, Lela Knox Shanks discovered many things she could do to help her husband. Many books have described ways to manage and improve the behaviors of Alzheimer's patients, but none surpasses what we discover here.

One of the keys to Lela Knox Shank's methods is that she allows her husband to be as independent as possible. This approach is good for both patients and their caregivers. Patients who are allowed to carry out daily activities such as dressing or bathing for as long as possible retain a sense of their own competence, and also struggle less with their caregivers. Lela Knox Shanks does not take over daily tasks for her husband but finds ways to modify the tasks or to help him get started on them. She developed remarkable strategies so that her husband could continue shaving, dressing, bathing, brushing his teeth. I was struck particularly by the simple and practical ways she modified her husband's wardrobe. To make it easier for him—or for her—to put on or take off his socks, she bought the most stretchable socks she could find. But because Hughes Hannibal Shanks had never worn casual clothes, she did not buy him sweatsuits, even though that would have made her job easier. In this and other examples we see the importance of making modifications but still respecting the patient's dignity and values. We also learn the importance of giving reassurance and affection to the Alzheimer's patient, rather than confronting him or getting angry over what he can't do. Lela Knox Shanks never treated her husband as someone who could not think or feel. Instead, she learned to recognize and validate his feelings, despite the distortions caused by his illness.

Another important theme in this book is that simple modifications in our homes and in our routines can make caregiving more manageable. We learn about some very interesting ways of modifying the home environment so that it is more supportive to someone with memory loss, and thus easier on the caregiver. My favorite example is the way Lela Knox Shanks helped her husband find his way to the bathroom at night by building a partition to guide him. Many caregivers who struggle with this problem can probably identify other simple and practical strategies that will help.

Besides these practical strategies and modifications, caregivers need something more in order to cope with the ongoing pressures they face—support and understanding from the people around them. Friends and family sometimes drift away from the caregiver, because they do not know what to say or do or because the care recipient's illness makes them uncomfortable. Lela Knox Shanks describes the support she received from her family and from some of the professionals she came in contact with. But she also created support for herself in support groups and through her other activities. We cannot take it for granted that caregivers will receive support. Too many are alone and cut off from people who could help. Their families don't understand, or just give advice, rather than listening or helping out in tangible ways. And too many professionals are not sufficiently knowledgeable or concerned about the problems that caregivers face.

Support also includes finding people to share some of the caregiving load. Lela Knox Shanks was fortunate to have located an adult day-care program suitable for her husband. Families sometimes wait too long to seek out this kind of help. In too many communities, however, appropriate services are not available or affordable. The United States is alone among the economically developed countries of the world in not having universal, publicly supported programs of care for the chronically disabled elderly. Looking at the enormous burden of care faced by familiies, we must ask how long it will be before our society recognizes the need to provide help on a consistent basis.

Families are often advised to get one particular type of help: that is, to put their relative in a nursing home. That advice may be hasty or mistaken for two reasons. First, physicians, social workers, and others who tell the family to institutionalize the patient often do not understand the options available to make home care more manageable. Lela Knox Shanks shows what can be done to keep an Alzheimer's patient at home. Many people may not choose or may be unable to do as much as she has done. But those who are determined to provide home care can do so, even in the face of severe and debilitating diseases. When caregivers want to provide care in the home, we should encourage and support them, not tell them they are making a mistake. Second, families are led to believe that nursing home placement will relieve their stress. In fact, however, institutionalization alters but does not eliminate stress. Caregivers who place the patient in a nursing home no longer have the strain associated with daily care tasks, but now they are visiting the facility, learning to interact with the staff, and giving up control over how their relative is cared for. There may also be increased feelings of guilt and greater family conflict over whether it was the right decision. And of course there is the burden of cost: families must find a way to pay for the nursing home, because chronic care is not covered by Medicare. There is no one answer to the question of placement. Certainly there should be no shame when a family must turn to a nursing home, because, as this book shows, the effort to keep an Alzheimer's patient at home can be enormous. But families need information so that they can make choices about care that are consistent with their values. And those who are willing to make sacrifices to keep someone at home also need support, including respite services such as adult day care.

In the final analysis, though, this book is about something larger than the sum of its parts. It is about love and commitment between a husband and wife. Lela Knox Shanks does not let Alzheimer's disease destroy her relationship or her memories. Instead, she finds new meaning and strength in her commitment. Everyone involved in the care of older people needs to read this book, and to be reminded that caregiving is a very personal and loving process.

Acknowledgments

This book was made possible by the giving spirit and generosity of our family, our friends, and total strangers.

My deep gratitude goes to Dell Smith and to Gordon Dickerson. Dell is our unofficially adopted son who showed up at our door in 1989 with a big box and announced, "I brought you a computer and a printer for all those books you are going to write." I was grateful but unimpressed, since I was a computer illiterate and this was my most stressful period with Hughes. The computer sat there. In 1990 Gordon Dickerson, one of Hughes's colleagues, called after hearing me speak on caregiving and suggested I write a book about Alzheimer's disease. I still did nothing. Gordon called back a year later and volunteered to take the manuscript to a publisher if I would write it. It was after his generous offer that I began to work on the book.

My deep gratitude also goes to Vivian Whipp and Cynthia Pemberton, who were with me from the beginning of this project, reading and editing the entire manuscript; to Leslie Whipp for editing and also for instructing me on how to get started in the first place; to Nan Graf for her help with the editing; and to Carole Smith, who always gave me a place to "crash" and to talk about the work. Many thanks also to Genie Logan, Loretta Russell, Leola Bullock, Jean Chicoine, Omell McMillan, Rita Schriner, Ann Gell, Ada Munson, and Naomi Hull for their support.

Grateful acknowledgments also go to the Thanks Be To Grandmother Winifred Foundation in Wainscott, New York, for the grant that helped pay Hughes's day-care costs while I worked on this project; to Jean Evans, Helen Brame, and Norma Larson for permitting me to include their stories; to Dr. Barry Reisberg, director of the Aging and Dementia Research Center, New York University Medical Center, for granting permission to include his Global Deterioration Scale.

I am indebted as well to Nancy Brown, Nebraska Division of Standards; Randy Musselman and the Ombudsmen Office of the Nebraska Department on Aging; Linda Stuart, On-Line Survey Certification and Reporting, Kansas City, Missouri; Sue Garrett and George Hiatt, who, like Dell Smith, came to my rescue when I had computer problems; the reference staff at the Bennett Martin Public Library, Don L. Love Library, and C. Y. Thompson Library in Lincoln, Nebraska. Special thanks to Sandy Bliss, Carol Kurtzhals, Deb Peck, Karen Noel, Barbara McCabe, and Barbara Sand, all of whom gave me a forum for presenting my caregiving approach in the earliest years. Thanks also to Florence Schlegelmilch and Dr. Samuel Lipkin.

I am deepy grateful to our children, Nena St. Louis, Cedric Shanks, Shela Omell Richards, and Eric Hughes Shanks, all of whom helped edit some part of the manuscript, and to their spouses, Michael Lewis, Chris Shanks, Jim Richards, and Sherry Waldman, who gave me support and encouragement to complete this project. A special thanks goes to Eric, who has been on call since his father's diagnosis of Alzheimer's disease.

Your Name Is Hughes Hannibal Shanks

Introduction

My husband, Hughes, has Alzheimer's disease.

Alzheimer's is an illness that leads to dementia. It shrinks the brain and destroys the ability of the mind to function "normally." Irreversible and deadly, it is the fourth leading cause of death in adults in the United States today. Estimates are that nearly 5 percent of the U. S. population over age sixty-five has severe dementia and another 10 percent has mild to moderate dementia. Alzheimer's disease "accounts for about half of all such cases."[1]

Hughes and I were enjoying a life of luxury, comfort, and pure leisure when he first showed signs of the disease in 1984. He was sixty-five, and I was fifty-seven. For the next two years, he had long periods—up to several months at a time—of lucidity, and then suddenly he would wake up in the morning and not know who I was. Finally, in 1986 he was given several tests, including a CAT scan of his brain and an electroencephalogram, which traces brain waves. The evaluating doctors, an internist and a neurologist, diagnosed his condition as multi-infarct dementia, a condition similiar to Alzheimer's disease but one of several different types of dementia. The doctors said he had probably suffered several small strokes over the years, damaging his brain irreparably; I could expect him to deteriorate mentally and physically over an indeterminable amount of time, until he became totally helpless and dependent. They said there was no cure and nothing they could do. As for medication, I was given the name of one drug, described as very expensive and very ineffective. We were sent home without any instructions, references, or suggestions as to how to proceed or where to go for help. I assumed that the doctors had provided me all the information they had available at the time.

In 1988 Hughes was evaluated by a second team of professionals: a psychiatrist, accompanied by a registered nurse, a social worker, and a pharmacist. After another round of interviews and tests, the diagnosis was Alzheimer's disease. Our youngest son, Eric—the only one of our children still living in the same state, was there, and we held on to each other when the diagnosis was given. Eric began to weep quietly. I had to be strong; I choked back the tears. They would come later, many times over the years.

This time, I was instructed to oversee Hughes's taking the medications previously prescribed (for his high blood pressure, among other things), to check our home for safety measures, and to stop Hughes from driving. I was also given four pamphlets, one on drugs and the others on hints for making the home environment safe for the patient with memory loss.

The bottom line of this evaluation was the same as the first, however: Hughes would eventually become totally helpless. I groped and grasped for another answer, entreating the doctors each time to say it wasn't so, that it might just be a big mistake after all, a misdiagnosis, as it were. But I was told this time as before that the various laboratory tests eliminated the possibility of a misdiagnosis. The results showed that Hughes had none of the common causes of a *reversible* dementia: no vitamin B_{12} or folic acid or thyroid deficiencies, no anemia, no infection. There was no mistake.

This second evaluation team emphasized many times how difficult it would be to take care of Hughes myself. I tried to solicit from the group some possibility of finding families who had had positive and successful experiences caring for Alzheimer's patients at home. That idea was not encouraged. I was given the name, phone number, time, and meeting place of the local chapter of the Alzheimer's Disease and Related Disorders Association; that was the most valuable information I received.[2] Once again we were sent home by professionals without any specific instructions on how to manage Hughes in our home. (I learned later that at that time only two of some three thousand physicians listed with the state medical association were specializing in geriatrics. I also learned that there were only fourteen schools in the United States offering postdoctoral residency in gerontology and geriatrics.)[3]

When we left the clinic, I realized that I was on my own. The clinicians could diagnose the disease but apparently had no knowledge of how one might successfully manage an Alzheimer's patient outside of an institution. As Eric drove us home, my mind whirled and turned on what I must do next. First, I must develop a plan for our survival—our creative survival. I thought, Alzheimer's could not be outside the human experience because Hughes is still a human being. I believed nothing could destroy anyone's essential humanness, and I knew there were no barriers between souls. Were we, the so-called normal ones, the smart ones, not evolved enough to figure out a way to accommodate our loved one in his own home? I knew deep inside that there had to be a way, although I had no clue as to what I would do or where to begin. I had scarcely even heard the word *Alzheimer's* beyond the fact that it was deadly. I was no stranger to adversity—I had been born into it—but I do not think anyone could be prepared to face this disease.

In retrospect, however, I recognize three major influences in my life that led me to believe it was possible to take care of Hughes and at the same time live my own life to the fullest: my African-American heritage; my relationship with my parents, especially the effect on me of my mother's death; and my spiritual development, which had been greatly influenced by two women, Sharon and Orpha, whom I refer to in the text as "the sisters" (see chapter 8).

From my heritage, I learned very early that there are some circumstances in our lives that for a time, at least, we cannot change. That was my reality as an African-American child growing up under legal racial segregation in the 1920s and 1930s. Adversity was always nearby for me and for my family. At the same time, I watched my strong mother defy racial segregation laws, gender taboos, and religious customs. She had a zest for life that even Jim Crow laws could not quell. She refused to be anything but a free spirit. She seemed to thrive on adversity and lived as if nothing were insurmountable. As a teenager, I was often embarrassed by her, and yet I admired her more than anyone. But I did not understand how she could take such risks, ignoring tradition and being such an individual.

Both she and my father had been my greatest sources of strength; even after I married Hughes, I still depended upon my mother for guidance and emotional support. I was not yet ready to grow up. But both my parents had died of cancer, three years apart, by the time I was thirty. I watched my mother in her last week of life as she lay bedfast, giving praise and thanksgiving for her life with her final labored breath. Even with open sores from her head to her feet, she never complained. Keeping a sense of humor to the end, she died as she had lived—with enthusiasm and grace. Clearly, she had something inside that transcended her physical or worldly condition, and at age twenty-seven I did not understand that. I wondered how she could give thanks when her body was covered in sores. What did she know about life that I did not know?

After the death of my parents, despite being a grown woman with a loving, supportive husband and three children, I felt all alone, like an orphan child. I experienced great pain, anger, and depression. They had been my props, and now that they were gone, I was anchorless. The outer world had failed me, and I began an internal search—for exactly what, I did not know, but I knew that my mother had had a faith and a knowledge of life that I had not yet experienced.

When I came out of the depression, I found myself on a new threshold of consciousness with a new sense of life and a new awareness of self, but my internal search was just beginning. I had not yet found what I was seeking. That would come later when I met the sisters. But the pain of losing my parents had given me an inner toughness I did not have before; by my thirty-first birthday I was determined never to be defeated by anything in my life.

That is why at the time of Hughes's diagnosis, when the clinicians predicted only doom and gloom for our future, I never believed them for one minute! The fact that this was the prevailing mind-set for Alzheimer's families meant nothing to me. Neither did I believe that Hughes had to spend the rest of his days living as a wretched victim. By the time we reached home, I was determined to find meaning and purpose and, especially, sanity in the midst of what the world calls "madness." I knew that as individuals we have a choice, that we get to decide how we shall internalize events in our lives. I knew that it was not the events that destroy us but how we choose to internalize them.

Today, twelve years since Hughes's first symptoms, we have reestablished stability and quality in our lives despite his continuing deterioration. I began a new career in 1989 as an independent scholar and lecturer, traveling when necessary, and speaking on African-American history, how women can achieve wholeness, the development of an inner life, and caregiving. I had to go to work to help pay for Hughes's new medical expenses. I had done public speaking nearly all my life but had never before been paid for it.

This book is about the choices I have made in my determination to take care of Hughes in our home (without giving him sedating or tranquilizing drugs) and at the same time to live my life to the fullest. None of this has been easy, but I have found it possible. As far back as I can remember, I was taught that the difficulty of a job is never a reason not to do it. As Eleanor Roosevelt said, "You must do the thing you think you cannot do."[4]

This book is written for both in-home caregivers and professional caregivers (including medical personnel), since the Alzheimer's patient may need both kinds of care. It is also for the policymakers who make critical monetary decisions that directly affect the quality and quantity of health care available to Hughes and other patients, and the level of research to find a cure. As a caregiver I discovered that I had to be also a researcher and a political advocate in order to give Hughes the best possible care, as well as to protect myself financially in case I survive him. It has taken several years of investigating numerous sources to gather the information I have needed to be a creative caregiver. I was never able to find everything I needed in one source alone. Neither was I able to find a single source that discussed in depth the humanness of the Alzheimer's patient along with the possibility that an in-home caregiver could have a positive and rewarding experience. Hence, I have tried to bring together in one place what I have learned and used to take care of Hughes and to take care of myself.

This material is presented in four parts. Part 1 gives Hughes's history as a patient, describes and explains the symptoms and the stages of Alzheimer's disease (AD), and shows why acceptance of the patient's humanness is crucial to good, creative care.

Part 2 describes techniques for the successful management of the patient in the home in each of the three stages. I discuss the question of violence and ways to deal with problem behavior, how to keep the patient clean, and my belief that it is possible for some AD patients to reach a level of competency even though living in the world of dementia.

Part 3 details twenty life skills for caregivers, from reinforcing one's own identity separate from the patient's to looking for small joys. I call these skills coping and survival strategies. It is here too that I tell about the two women, the sisters, who helped me find what I had been searching for all my life.

Part 4 discusses the future for AD patients and caregivers. Chapter 10 provides the latest information available at the time of this writing about scientific research and assistive technology; describes the changes in some nursing homes from the medical model to the social model—including the development of special-care units—and the positive effects of those changes for AD patients; and explores changes in public policy that could affect the patient and the caregiver. The last chapter is about sexuality, the new life of the caregiver, and the rewards of caregiving.

Because everything in this book is interconnected, each part interlaps and overlaps with the other parts. Much of the care of an AD patient is about repetition; therefore, some information is repeated in order to tell the story. Interspersed throughout the book is some of the history of Hughes's life, my life, and our lives together. Who was he before AD? What did he stand for? What did his life mean? The appendix presents excerpts from some of his writings over a forty-year period. I believe they give insight into Hughes the man, the husband, the father, the fighter, the friend—the *person* who I believe is still present underneath the dementia. The appendix also includes my outline for a possible training course for caregivers. It ends with essays written by our children to express how they feel about their father's having Alzheimer's disease.

Hughes may now be in some part of the final stage—I am not sure. Each day brings more brain deterioration and some strange new behavior. But when I treat Hughes like a human being and go with the flow of life, I find the strength to face each new obstacle, a solution for each new problem. Difficulties can be transcended. There is always a new way. The choice is ours.

PART ONE
The Symptoms and Stages of Alzheimer's Disease

ONE

How Alzheimer's Started in Hughes

The first time Hughes showed definite signs of Alzheimer's disease was a night in August 1984. We were driving home to Lincoln, Nebraska, after visiting our son Cedric and his family in La Grande, Oregon.

We were both retired and had begun to travel. We loved taking long car trips together. We liked the closeness and the intimacy of car travel. We liked each other. We enjoyed being together.

Hughes had retired from the Social Security Administration in 1976 after more than thirty years of federal service, including post office employment and active military duty during World War II. But for most of those years he had worked as a claims representative, interviewing clients who applied for Social Security benefits. He was a skilled interviewer and enjoyed his work. He liked the one-on-one contact with the public. He loved working for the people. He also liked solving problems, especially difficult cases where eligibility for benefits was hard to prove. It was always a moment of joy for him when he found the missing piece of evidence that established eligibility for the client. He saw himself as an advocate for the people, a true public servant.

Hughes's job was not an easy one, however. In addition to the high level of technical difficulty of the position itself, he worked under the constant pressure and stress of institutionalized racism. In the 1950s, when he was hired by the Social Security Administration, racial segregation and discrimination were still legal in the United States, taken for granted as part of the American way of life. Actually, the term "institutionalized racism" had scarcely been defined, much less acknowledged. But racial prejudice and racial discrimination were the reality for African-Americans in every aspect of their daily lives.

Under these circumstances, especially as the first Black person to be hired in his office, Hughes walked a tightrope. He faced and fought racial discrimination of all kinds throughout his years with the federal government.[1] I am sure this took its toll; stress always takes its toll. Amazingly, he often appeared able to let the bitterness go, but when the injustices got to him, he would break down and cry. Nevertheless, he still loved his work, and he was rewarded with job satisfaction and self-fulfillment. Wherever we went, clients came up to him, reintroducing themselves and expressing gratitude for his efforts on their behalf. He took their attention in stride, saying he was just doing his job.

In the 1960s when computers were installed in his office, Hughes hated them. He said they took the human element out of his work, and he felt he could no longer serve the people. He was a realist and accepted that computers were here to stay, but he said he now felt in the way and that it was time to move on. Hughes had expressed over the years the importance of knowing when we had outlived our usefulness in any position in life. He always said nobody was indispensable. He was never afraid of making a change. Once the computers were in, we began planning his exit. He was a claims analyst when he retired.

With some effort, we got it all worked out: I would find a job when Hughes retired, since our youngest child, Eric, was still in high school. We had helped our other three children pay for college, and we wanted to be financially able to give Eric the same support.

Hughes had never before accepted the idea of my working outside the home, and this had been a major source of unresolved conflict between us throughout our marriage. I came from a long line of strong-willed, independent-thinking women who never looked to their spouses, the government, or anyone else for their support. They looked to themselves. My mother had held a job forever. During the Great Depression, when most people could find no work, Mama had two jobs. Her mother worked until forced to retire because of her age.

Hughes, on the other hand, was one of twelve children whose mother had never worked outside the home. He told me many times, "I don't want my babies going out in the cold for a babysitter to raise. A family needs someone at home for backup and support at all times." There would be no latchkey children in our household if he had anything to do with it. I had been a latchkey child and knew well the potential dangers and the often accompanying neglect. I didn't want latchkey children either, but I was clearly torn. When I graduated magna cum laude with a journalism degree in 1949, staying home taking care of four babies and a stepson was not exactly what I had in mind. Ever since I could remember, I had expected to be a newspaperwoman. I wanted a career, not to mention the additional income we needed.

Over the years, however, whenever I talked of going to work, Hughes just got one more part-time job. At one time he had three part-time jobs in addition to his full-time position. In those years he would wake up from a short nap and ask, "Where do I go now?" Not until 1975 did he reluctantly agree to my taking a job. I think he realized there was no stopping me now.

During the seven years I worked outside the home, he took over all the housekeeping responsibilities. He was an excellent cook when we got married—in fact, he taught me how to cook—so there was always good, warm food waiting for me when I came home from work. He tried hard to be supportive of me in every way, but it was extremely difficult for him to accept not having me at home and at his every whim, as in the past. (I say this not negatively but as a simple fact.) Looking back, I realize that it was during the years I worked that I began to notice his personality change, and personality change is one of the first slow and subtle symptoms of AD.[2]

Of course, not knowing anything about the disease at that time, I did not connect these changes in Hughes to AD as we drove along that night in 1984. We were about six hours from Lincoln, both tired but basking in the good times we had shared with Cedric and our daughter-in-law, Chris, and our grandchildren, Carrie and Christopher. Hughes was driving, and suddenly he called me Nena, our older daughter's name. Our younger daughter is Shela and my name is Lela; since all our names sound so much alike, I paid no attention at first. But he continued to repeat the mistake. Finally, I asked him, "Why do you keep calling me Nena?" He seemed oblivious to my voice, as if he had not heard me. And then he said, "How are the kids doing in the back seat?" Since our "baby," Eric, was twenty-six, I knew something was wrong. I thought to myself, "He has gone out of his mind." I felt I had to act quickly, and I ordered him to pull over to the shoulder and stop. We exchanged places, and as I began driving, his speech rambled. I felt terrified and started praying, not knowing what to expect next.

He dozed a bit, but at one point he tried to open the door and get out of the car. He said he was tired and was going upstairs to bed. With all the authority in me, I screamed, "Don't you dare touch that seatbelt or try to get up!" That got his attention. He calmed down and dozed restlessly the remainder of the trip home.

We arrived in town about two in the morning. The streets were well lighted, but as we drove down the main street, Hughes said, "This is not Lincoln! You have gone to the wrong town!" He continued to fume that I had brought us to the wrong place until I pulled into our driveway. The moment we arrived home, however, he was himself again, with no recollection at all of anything he had said or done in the past six hours. He proceeded to unpack the car methodically as he always did after a trip. It was back to business as usual for him, but not for me. After that night our lives would never be the same again.

TWO
The Three Stages of the Disease

After Hughes's first diagnosis in 1986, I began reading about strokes and memory loss; after his second diagnosis, I began seriously studying about Alzheimer's disease. I learned that one assessment tool used to describe the stages of AD is the Global Deterioration Scale (GDS) developed by Dr. Barry Reisberg.[1] This scale, capsulized in table 1, describes seven stages that show how the AD patient's progression in the disease retraces in reverse the development of a child. There is hardly universal agreement on the number of stages, however, or where one ends and another begins.[2] Neither are there clear lines of demarcation between what have been called "tiers" within each stage, marking the progression of the disease from the beginning to the end of a given stage. I have never met a physician who would speak to me specifically on the stages of the disease, probably because so little is still known about AD and also because the fluctuation and unpredictability of the symptoms make the disease individualized in each patient. The symptoms and the length of time spent in any one stage may vary from patient to patient.[3]

But even though medical professionals shy away from talking about stages, caregivers do not. I have never met a caregiver who did not speak in terms of stages. In order to keep going day in and day out, caregivers need some sense of where the patient is in the progression of the disease—even if they are wrong. Thinking in terms of stages helps them better understand the patient's behavior and what solutions may be possible. Since the doctors did not help me, I had to figure out the stages for myself, and I am relating them here as they applied to Hughes.

I observed three broad stages, as have numerous long-term, in-home caregivers I have talked to.[4] They are the first or beginning stage, the second or middle stage, and the third or terminal stage. I also found that each stage has at least two tiers, although they are nebulous and often difficult to pin down. Throughout all stages and tiers, however, two symptoms have affected Hughes's overall behavior, despite the fluctuation and unpredictability of the disease. These are confusion and disorientation, both due to the patient's gradual loss of memory.[5]

The onset of the symptoms is so slow and so insidious that major personality changes are well in place before the family or the patient understands the reasons for them.[6] The two years between Hughes's memory

Table 1   Reisberg's Global Deterioration Scale

Reisberg's scale describes how Alzheimer's disease's pattern parallels in reverse that of child development—and tells doctors and relatives what to expect next of Alzheimer's victims.

Approx. Age	Abilities Acquired	Alzheimer's Stage	Abilities Lost
12+ years	Hold a job	Borderline	Hold a job
7–12 years	Handle simple finances	Early	Handle simple finances
5–7 years	Select proper clothes	Moderate	Select proper clothes
5 years	Put on clothes	Severe	Put on clothes
4 years	Shower unaided		Shower unaided
4 years	Go to toilet unaided		Go to toilet unaided
3–4½ years	Control urine		Control urine
2–3 years	Control bowels		Control bowels
15 months	Speak five or six words	Late	Speak five or six words
1 year	Speak one word		Speak one word
1 year	Walk		Walk
6–9 months	Sit up		Sit up
2–3 months	Smile		Smile

Source: M. Roach, "Reflection in a Fatal Mirror," in *Aging*, E. C. Goldstein, ed. Vol. 2, Art. 83 (Boca Raton FL: Social Issues Resource Series, 1981).

lapse in 1984 and his first diagnosis in 1986 were probably the most maddening years of my life. I was angry at least 75 percent of the time, yelling and screaming at my husband, wondering what was happening to this man I had loved so much for so many years. Hughes had been my college sweetheart, my one and only. We had met in 1946 in college. I was nineteen, and he was twenty-seven. Now, after almost forty years together, I watched helplessly as he turned into someone I did not know. Outwardly, he still looked the same. His physical bearing did not change, but his behavior became different and unpredictable. I was totally baffled. I did not like this person he was becoming. It was as if he had regressed to adolescence. I thought he was turning into a weakling, and my great attraction to Hughes in the first place had been his fearlessness, his self-confidence, his strong character. He had always acted so much like a man!

The first man in my life, my father, had by his own admission never been a match for my mother's ambition, vision, and ego. Mama, with only an eighth-grade education, thought she could do anything! Papa, a quiet, gentle, warm man, was equally educated and much better read. But having lived his entire life under American apartheid, when "uppity" Black men were lynched for talking back, Papa had been beaten down by racial segregation and prejudice. He knew "his place" and he stayed in it. Hughes was different. He would not accept that "place." He was a fighter and a rebel, a risk taker; he represented the manhood I had been looking for.

I was a country girl from Green Pastures, Oklahoma, a place not even on the map. I was as green as the pastures. Hughes was big-city streetwise. He had grown up in St. Louis, hawking newspapers on the streets when he was only eight years old. At sixteen he graduated from high school in the midst of the Great Depression. He had always dreamed of going to college. His parents had met at Philander Smith College in Little Rock, Arkansas, after the turn of the century. They had instilled in Hughes and in all their twelve children a deep appreciation for books and reading, learning and higher education. But college for him in 1936 was out of the question. There were no jobs and no money.

Hughes always disputed the claim that anybody who wanted work could find it. He knew better. His inability to find a job in his hometown during the Depression left a bitterness in him he never forgot. In 1938, he was a young husband with a wife and a new son, Ron, and no job to support his young family. In desperation he left home with five dollars and hopped a freight train to Chicago to look for work. Relatives took him in, but those were hard times. He told the story of once having to choose between paying his rent or going to the dentist. He paid his rent, and when the pain in his mouth became unbearable, he pulled his aching tooth out with pliers. Eventually, he got steady work as a painter's apprentice. But that separation ended his first marriage.

When Pearl Harbor was bombed in 1941, Hughes was one of the first volunteers. Initially, however, he was sent back home and told there was no place for him in his country's army; he would have to wait until a segregated unit was formed. Hughes was not discouraged, though. He was determined. Despite the prejudice and the legal discrimination, he felt this was still his country, the only country he had or knew, and he wanted to serve. He also wanted the adventure—and he got it. When his ship was torpedoed in the Pacific, he was injured and adrift on a raft for some days before being rescued (the story as he told it in verse is included in the appendix). He came home a hero in 1945, decorated with a Purple Heart.

After the war ended, the GI Bill made college possible for Hughes and thousands of poor veterans like him; he enrolled in the summer of 1946. Immediately, he joined the drama club, the Stagecrafters, and earned the role of Grandpa Vanderhot in the Moss Hart and George S. Kaufman play *You Can't Take It with You*. We met that fall in the drama club. I think I knew even before our first date that I wanted to marry him. The first time we danced our bodies came together as if we had been rehearsing for that moment all our lives. I do not think he knew what was happening. He said my youth and boldness frightened him. All I knew was that he was the man I wanted. My mother was alarmed and came to Kansas City to meet Hughes while we were touring with a play. She gave us a qualified blessing, saying, "I guess he is all right." The next year we eloped. Married students were considered a bad influence in those days, so we continued to live apart in our dormitories and kept our marriage secret for the rest of the semester.

Coming from two entirely different backgrounds, we had many differences throughout all the years of our marriage but I never ever contemplated divorce. It was as if Hughes and I were a part of each other, belonged together. Couples who separated after thirty-five and forty years of marriage had always puzzled me. But as Hughes began to change (before I knew he had AD), I thought maybe this was why: because one spouse turned into a completely different person. I began to think the unthinkable: had I married the wrong man after all? It was almost a relief to learn at his first diagnosis that Hughes was in the beginning stage of dementia.

FIRST STAGE

The first stage of the disease could be called the "denial" stage, for both the patient and the family, since the patient in the beginning is still able to take care of all his or her personal needs and generally to continue living a normal life. In fact the patient is often well into the first stage of the disease before the family knows anything is wrong. Yet all the while these early symptoms are stealthily creeping in, changing the personality of the patient. For example, in the first tier of the first stage, Hughes was completely able to take care of himself. In the second tier he began to need some assistance. By the third tier he had forgotten entirely how to initiate bathing and dressing.

Also in the first tier he knew me 99 percent of the time. In fact, it was two years from his first memory lapse in 1984 to the next time, in 1986, when he did not know who I was. By then he was in the second tier and often called me an impostor. Two years later, in the third tier, he called me "sir" and usually thought I was a man. By the end of the first stage he needed twenty-four-hour care. I believe he spent five or six years in the first stage.

The early signs of AD in Hughes were these subtle but far-reaching personality changes.

INDECISION

Hughes had always been able to make a decision on the spot. He could think through everything in an instant and never waver from his decision. I was the indecisive one. I needed time to consider all options and alternatives. I wanted to weigh every detail involved. Hughes acccpted decision-making as a natural part of his responsibility as a man, as a husband and father. Throughout the years of our marriage I had been quite willing to lean on him, and also to let him take the heat if a decision proved to be a poor one. Consequently, when he suddenly could not make a decision, I knew something was wrong. This wasn't the same person I had married. I looked for answers everywhere—except, of course, to AD. Wondering whether people naturally changed like this as they aged, I researched the aging process extensively and discovered this was not part of normal aging. I tried not to worry, but as his indecisiveness increased, I gradually had to take on more and more of the family decision-making. In the beginning I resented it deeply. My nice, warm, protective cocoon was falling apart.

INSECURITY

Hughes's fears began to equal his indecisiveness. He was like a child afraid to be alone. He had always been possessive, but the way he clung to me now, never wanting me out of his sight, was different.

SILLINESS

Hughes had always been pleasant and friendly, but his demeanor was dignified and serious. Now he laughed at everything and made ridiculous comments totally out of character for him. When I asked, "What is the matter with you?" his stock answer was, "Who? Me?" He never really seemed to understand what I was talking about, probably because he had already forgotten the question.

SPONTANEOUS WEEPING

As his personality continued to change, weeping became a daily ritual for Hughes.[7] When he was not laughing inappropriately, he was weeping spontaneously. Though I had admired him for not being too proud and too macho to cry, he had done so infrequently—perhaps four or five times throughout our marriage—but now he broke down every day, anywhere, at any time, in front of anyone. When asked why he was crying, he always shook his head like a little child and said sadly, "I don't know."

PROGRESSIVE MEMORY LOSS

The best-known early symptom of AD is short-term memory loss.[8] Hughes could remember events from fifty years ago in great detail, but he could not recall what had happened five minutes earlier. As the disease progresses, patients lose both short-term and long-term memory. The first things they learned in life are the last things they forget.

But memory loss was not the first symptom I had noticed in Hughes. He was known in our family for his absentmindedness. He could read the newspaper, hold a conversation, and never remember a word said. Our daughter Nena called him the "Space Cadet." When confronted with his nonattentiveness, he explained that in growing up with eleven siblings there had never been a place or a time at home when he could be alone. To compensate, he had learned to make a solitary place inside himself by shutting off all sounds from the outside world.

In my denial, oh, how I wanted to believe that his memory lapses were due to his known spaciness. But the lapses continued unabated. There was no denying that all our fights centered on something he forgot. He would drop me off somewhere and forget to pick me up. When I asked why, he disclaimed any knowledge of where I had been and accused me of leaving without telling him. Or we would agree on a major purchase, but when I followed through, he accused me of not consulting him.

These misunderstandings were soon happening not once a day but all through the day. There were moments when I questioned my own sanity. I remembered a woman living in the same apartment building during the early years of our marriage who thought her husband was trying to convince her she was crazy. I began to wonder, "Is this what Hughes is trying to do to me?" Remember, he still looked the same, and in the first stage the patient is often in and out of the disease. I bought notebooks and slates for home and car use and started writing down our daily schedules. I insisted each day that we go over our schedules together, then that we each sign the other's schedule, complete with date and time. In only a few days it became clear that I was not crazy. Hughes was losing his short-term memory.

CONFUSION AND DISORIENTATION

Everything was beginning to look different to Hughes—people, places, and things—because of his memory loss. I realize now that he was in a state of increasing confusion and disorientation—symptoms that seem to go hand in hand—for many years before I knew he had the disease. In the first tier he often commented in passing that someone or some place or some object did not look the same. But when he reached the second tier, he would suddenly stop the car in the middle of the street, protesting, "That building doesn't belong over there!" In the third tier he could still drive, but I would have to tell him how to find his way.

In his growing confusion all his home chores took longer and longer for him to perform. Tasks involving several steps became overwhelming. By the time I took over Hughes's personal care, he needed four hours to go through the motions of preparing himself for bed.

As the family cook, Hughes had always prepared our holiday dinners. Our children loved his gourmet dishes; he was by far the better cook. But I began to notice he could no longer complete the preparations for a big or even a small family dinner. Cooking required too many steps and too many sequences. The last time Hughes tried to cook, he emptied an ice tray in a skillet on the stove and turned the burner up full blast.

WITHDRAWAL FROM FAMILY GATHERINGS

When Hughes began walking out on his family, we were puzzled and disconcerted. Before AD he had been a main player if not the center of every lively discussion taking place at our special family dinners. We often had three different debates going at one time, always controversial with loud, dogmatic voices for every side. Hughes was usually the family radical, not our children. But when he was no longer able to prepare the big dinners, he withdrew from the rest of the family.[9] We would find him in the basement, puttering among his wood pieces, trying to remember how he once put them together to make picture frames.

SECOND STAGE

The second stage of AD could be called the "aggression and hostility" stage. By this time, patients usually know they are no longer within their own control, and they may react by striking out in anger and violence at the caregiver. One can hardly fathom their inner agony in this stage! In a sense, they are in limbo: they are unable to take care of themselves, but they have not yet learned how to let others take care of them. Nor are they able to contribute to the relationship with their caregivers in the customary and usual sense. The beginning of this stage is probably the most critical time for determining whether the caregiver will keep the patient in the home or seek out a long-term care facility.

This stage, beginning in 1988 or 1989, was by far the most difficult for me. I was still learning about the disease and did not know what to expect. Every day Hughes would exhibit some new and bizarre behavior that I had never encountered before. One minute he might be friendly and the next minute hostile. I was never really sure whether he would hurt me or not. There were times that I didn't know when I could eat, when I could sleep, when I could bathe, or when I could use the bathroom. Looking back, I believe that competent training in patient management techniques would have helped me get through this stage with much less stress (see chapter 10 and the appendix).

The second stage for Hughes was marked by an escalation of some first-stage symptoms: continuing memory loss, confusion and disorientation, withdrawal from family gatherings (which became so complete that most family members began to avoid such gatherings, without openly saying so). His indecision, insecurity, silliness, and spontaneous weeping, however, were replaced by hostility. This and other symptoms developed during the second stage.

AGITATION AND HOSTILITY

As Hughes lost more and more of his memory and thus became more and more confused and disoriented, he grew agitated and then angry. Undoubtedly, one symptom ignited another. In the beginning of this stage he sometimes projected his hostility and frustration on me.[10] The only time he became physically aggressive, however, was the day in 1988 when we returned home after receiving his second diagnosis: that is, the Alzheimer's diagnosis.

I was in the kitchen drawing a glass of water. Hughes came into the room and ordered me to put the glass down. Then he shouted, "Get out of this house! You are an impostor trying to break up my marriage!"[11] Suddenly, he reached for my gold necklace and broke it off my neck. I was not hurt, but I was afraid, not knowing what he might do next. I ran out the back door and sat in the sun. I did not have time to get my coat, and it was March and still cold. I cried and moaned, praying for an answer to what to do. After about twenty or thirty minutes, I tapped lightly on the back door. Hughes opened the door and expressed great relief that I was all right. He said, "Where have you been? I looked all over for you! I was just getting ready to call the police and report you as missing."

SUSPICION, ACCUSATIONS, AND PARANOIA

Showing how one symptom feeds into another, Hughes was suspicious of everyone, especially me; whenever he was suspicious, he followed up with an accusation; and his increasing mistrust of all those around him soon began to resemble paranoia.[12]

His accusations and suspicions of me in the first tier of the second stage had to do with events that were plausible: that is, events that could physically have occurred. But, to illustrate the tier-to-tier progression, by the time he had progressed to the third, the events his mind concocted had become bizarre and impossible. For example, in the first tier of the second stage Hughes was still driving and would sometimes drop me off at the front door of the federal building, where I would meet my friend Loretta for lunch. When I returned home, he would accuse me of having gone right through the building and out the back exit to meet my "boyfriend." While that was untrue, it was physically possible. But as he progressed to the second tier, his accusations were no longer even logical. Once, during our swimming class at the YWCA, I got out of the pool to use the bathroom. When I returned in moments, he accused me of going to meet my "boyfriend" in the women's locker room! By the third tier, he accused me of letting my boyfriend live in our home. After those accusations I could no longer deny that Hughes was losing the use of his rational mind.

He also became suspicious of our children, our closest friends, and especially meter readers and repairmen who came into our home. Even in the first stage he had accused Eric, our son, of taking his tools from the basement without permission and never returning them. By the second stage he had progressed to accusing every meter reader who came into the basement of stealing his tools, even after watching each one with an eagle eye from the time they entered until they left. After our plumber of twenty years had made a repair, Hughes went to his office and asked him if he had taken specific tools from our basement. The plumber had no idea what Hughes was talking about.

HIDING OBJECTS

Most irritating of all the symptoms for me as a careprovider was the habit Hughes developed of hiding things. Each morning we started the day by looking for essential personal items he had hidden: his shoes, pants, toothbrush, razor, eyeglasses, keys, dental bridge. Even before the AD was diagnosed we had had to replace his dental bridge twice, at $400 per replacement.

Whenever he could not find something, he would ask me, "Where did you put my shoes?" (or whatever), always adamant that either Eric or I had taken his possessions. In those days my first response was to try to reason with him. But one cannot reason with dementia. Often Hughes's hiding places suggested the dubious genius of a magician. At one time, Eric and I challenged each other to find his newest hiding place. His favorite spot, however, always remained the most obvious: under the mattress.

HALLUCINATIONS

Hughes had begun to see things that were not there as early as 1987.[13] He would ask me questions about "the child" that was with us; he thought a little boy or girl was eating at our table. Sometimes he thought we had a baby in the bed between us. Once he refused to come into the house "because that bad dog was in there barking." He also asked me if I had put the cat out, but we had not had a cat or any other animal for several years. His hallucinations became accusatory when he was sure I was letting "those men live in our basement." In his mind, these imaginary men were always my boyfriends. He often lectured and reprimanded me for "my shameful and immoral behavior." He once told me, "You should be ashamed of yourself, bringing those men in here right up under my nose." It was hard to stay calm and to stop trying to convince Hughes that he was wrong.

REPETITIVE ACTS

When Hughes would ask the same question over and over and over, he never understood my irritation with him, since he had already forgotten that he had asked the question before.[14] He also hummed the same tune repeatedly, hour after hour, day in and day out. He would get dressed in the morning, then put on another layer of clothes and sometimes a third, oblivious to the previous layer. There were periods when he was disoriented in time and got up in the middle of the night, dressing and undressing again and again. Since an AD patient has no short-term memory, he or she can repeat any such action indefinitely. It is as if something in the brain is stuck, like a needle on a record. Chris Milne, who became Hughes's psychologist, told me that the symptom of repetitive acts is called "perseveration."

SUNDOWNING

A daily event every evening after supper was Hughes's frantic pacing back and forth from the front door to the back door, hour after hour, locking and unlocking all doors while mumbling to himself. He seemed driven, compelled, unable to stop himself. He pulled the shades down and closed the drapes long before dark. He checked and rechecked all the windows, making sure they were locked, continuing to mumble anxiously. He would always be highly agitated, though he seldom paid any attention to me unless I tried to interfere. According to some AD experts, this symptom called "sundowning" has something to do with the absence of light.[15] I had known nothing of it until Hughes first began his nightly pacing.

WANDERING

One of the few symptoms I had heard of when Hughes was diagnosed with AD was the patient's tendency to wander. At the time Hughes began to exhibit this tendency, he was having frequent bouts of dizziness, which caused his gait to be unsteady; in addition, he was becoming increasingly incoherent. To a casual observer on the streets he could have easily been mistaken for an old man too drunk to find his way home. I was terrified that he might wander off and be picked up by the police; we had both grown up avoiding contact with the police like the plague. I expressed my fears to our son Cedric, who is in law enforcement. When he came to visit in 1989, he went to the police department with my concerns. Afterward, the captain of our district called and assured me that Hughes would be treated with respect and care.

Hughes wandered away from the day-care center two or three times. He was still so agile that he simply put one hand on the fence and vaulted to the other side. Fortunately, the day-care staff spotted him walking away each time and brought him back. Eventually, the center erected a higher barrier. Then Hughes pulled a chair up to the fence, but he was stopped by the staff before he could climb over.

In the summer of 1991 Hughes wandered off from home for the first time. He was sitting in the glider on our screened front porch when I went to the basement to put a load of clothes in the washer; when I returned, he was nowhere in sight. I was terrified! Only recently an elderly patient who wandered off from one of our local hospitals had been found dead the next morning in a drainage ditch. This could happen to Hughes! I had to find him. Our son Eric was at work, but his wife, Sherry, was home. She took one part of our neighborhood to search and I took the other. After alerting our neighbors and local businesses, I tried to think as I thought he would. I decided that he would either go where he saw children or follow the route we often took on our neighborhood walks. That is exactly what he had done. Like a homing pigeon, he had taken our usual walk and had stopped at our turnaround point, but he did not know how to come back. I found him trying to get into a parked car in which a puzzled-looking man at the wheel had locked the doors. I explained and apologized to the man. Hughes was very confused, and of course, he did not know me; it took a while to coax him to get into our car. Nevertheless, spotting Hughes that day was one of the happiest moments of my life.

INABILITY TO COMMUNICATE VERBALLY

From being unable to remember a specific word that he needed, Hughes next could not remember whole phrases or even his thought. Today, he talks infrequently, and when he does it is mostly gibberish. Occasionally, however, he will speak a short phrase or sentence that makes complete sense. For example, he sometimes says: "Okay," "Damn!" (if I touch him with cold hands), or "Get off my foot." One year ago he could still say, "Thank you," "I love you," "You do a good job."

INABILITY TO READ OR TO WRITE HIS NAME

Because Hughes loved reading and writing—in fact, he was once a teacher for the Laubach Literacy Training Program—it was heartbreaking to see these skills disappear. I believe he still recognizes individual words, but his memory is so impaired that he cannot remember to continue to the next word. His attention span compares to that of a year-old baby. He has been unable to write even his name for about three years.

DIZZINESS

The only physical problem Hughes showed as he has progressed in the disease was dizziness. It occurred most often when he first got up in the morning or when he stood up after some time in a sitting position. His physician prescribed meclizine, which has controlled that symptom to date.

CHILLINESS

Throughout all four seasons, Hughes complained of being cold. No matter how hot it was outside or inside, he was still cold, and his body also felt cold to the touch. Although this may have had something to do with the slower circulatory system of age, his physician explains that it may also have been caused by changes in his brain.

RETURN TO THE ORAL STAGE

Hughes at this writing will try to put anything in his mouth and eat it. Our bathroom has been stripped of toiletries for the last four or five years.

He has tried to drink his shaving lotion. He has eaten soap, tissues, raw pasta, lint, houseplants, and pieces of nutshells. When I am shaving him, he often reaches out with his lips for any object touching him around his mouth.

INCONTINENCE

Hughes began wearing protective briefs in 1992. His incontinence, probably the most dreaded of all symptoms for careproviders, started when he was no longer able to recognize the bathroom or to find his way to it in the house where we had lived for almost thirty years. Sometimes, he is *in* the bathroom and still looking for it. On more than one occasion he mistook the floor heat vent, the washbasin, or the bathtub for the commode. He has always shown a recognition of the stimulus to eliminate, but he no longer knows exactly what to do about it. He usually gives a clue to careproviders, however, by standing up suddenly and moving about. At least half the time, he makes some effort to help himself within his limited mental abilities.

INABILITY TO RECOGNIZE FAMILY MEMBERS

After the first incident in 1984 when Hughes did not know me, two years passed before it happened again—and again, he was out of his familiar home environment. We had traveled with the Nebraskans for Peace to a march in Washington DC. Hughes was lucid on the bus trip and also on the march, but by nightfall he no longer knew who I was. We were staying in the basement of a church in Maryland, and we had to take the subway and a cab to get back to the church. After I purchased the subway tokens, Hughes lost his and had to jump over the turnstile in order to catch the train.

We were preparing to bed down in our sleeping bags when suddenly Hughes turned on me, saying as before that I was an impostor trying to break up his marriage. Once again I was terrified, since we were so far from home and only one other person had returned to the church with us, a young woman who had become ill after the march. He was also more hostile and aggressive than I had ever seen him in our marriage. As his verbal attacks escalated, there were moments when I thought he was advancing on me. We were quartered in the Sunday School section, so I stacked tables and chairs between us. For a brief moment I was so afraid that I even contemplated calling the police, but I quickly dismissed that idea.

Suddenly I realized that if I believed my faith was real, then I had the protection of the universe right there in the room with me. I was aware immediately that only my fear could defeat me—not Hughes. Almost instinctively, I began to pray, believing that I would be given what I needed to get through this experience. Instantly, my feelings of terror subsided, and I could see that Hughes, even in a deranged state, was not bigger than God or life. I was guided to stay away from him, to keep quiet and not become involved with his comments but to continue with my preparations for bed and to center myself in prayer. Hughes harangued and rambled for about two hours before he finally settled down and zipped himself up in his sleeping bag. That night I tried to sleep with one eye open.

The next day, Ron and his daughter Stacey, Hughes's son and grand-daughter, came from Camden, New Jersey, to spend the afternoon with us as did our daughter Shela and her future husband, Jim, from New York City. Throughout their visit, Hughes did not recognize Ron. On our return trip home he was confused but cooperative.

Slowly and reluctantly, I began to see a pattern. Hughes was showing a significant loss of memory when he was out of his home environment, a loss he would never regain. Yet against my better judgment, I made one last trip with him. In 1987 we took Amtrak to New York City for the birth of Shela's second son, Zenith. We had driven to New York in 1982 when Shela's older son, Orpheus, was born. In 1987 she was in denial about her father's condition and pleaded with me to come. Hughes made the train trip to New York without difficulty, but once there he did not recognize Shela or her husband. "If that is Shela, why is she masquerading as some-body else?" he asked me, and, "If that is Shela, why is she going incognito?"

In my own denial, I was determined to take Hughes with me to see a Broadway play. Our daughter, of course, was recovering from childbirth, and our son-in-law had to go to work, so Hughes and I went by cab to the theater to see James Earl Jones in the Tony-award-winning play *Fences*. Hughes was obviously confused, but he managed to act as if he belonged there and knew what was going on; AD patients are often able "to maintain a facade of acceptable behavior."[16] Afterward, I thought it would be nice to see something of New York on foot, but that was a mistake. It was a mir-acle that I was able to find our way back to Shela and Jim's home. We fi-nally took the bus, transferring twice, and in those crowds I realized I had to keep my hands on Hughes at all times.

Our return trip to Lincoln was the worst experience of my life. Hughes thought he was on a ship instead of a train, and he not only did not know me but spent the last eight hours of the trip going from coach to coach, try-ing to run away from me. As bewildered passengers looked on, all I could do was chase after him, praying for guidance and hoping he would recognize me. Whenever he got tired of running, he sat in any empty seat, including the conductor's. I explained to the train attendant that my husband had AD. She understood and shared some harrowing experiences with demented patients traveling alone.

When the train finally arrived in Lincoln, Hughes refused to get off. But suddenly, like guardian angels, three passengers appeared out of nowhere to block all aisles and entries, leaving only the exit open to Hughes. Hughes looked at them and said, "Well, you are all against me," and got off the train. I looked for Eric, who had promised to pick us up, but he was nowhere in sight. Meanwhile, Hughes wrapped his arms around one of the columns on the station platform and refused to let go. I stood there feeling helpless, silly, and self-conscious as I tried unsuccessfully to pry his hands and arms loose.

All of a sudden, we saw some old friends rushing to board the train. Hughes recognized them and immediately put his arms to his sides and smiled, greeting our friends in a perfectly normal way. I seized that moment to pull him into the station, still hoping to see Eric (I learned later that he had forgotten). As we entered the station, Hughes thought I was Eric, and asked, "Where is your truck?" What luck, I thought. I told him it was up the street and encouraged him to follow me. He trailed behind, mumbling as we walked about three blocks to a hotel where we found a cab and came home. Once we were in our house, Hughes knew who I was again and asked, "Where is that boy I was with?" I tried to tell him that I was the boy, but he was not convinced. He went outside in the dark and walked around the house looking for that boy. I made up my mind that no matter who was born or who died, I would never again take Hughes, by myself, far from his home environment.

After that trip Hughes still had some periods of lucidity, and he began to realize that he had not known Shela on our visit. He wrote two letters to her that he never mailed but tucked away in his drawer.

Dear Shela:
You were, without doubt, the first person to be touched with my memory loss. But you are not the only member of our family whom I often call by an incorrect name. Please forgive me for the times I thought you were someone else. But I was acting what my mind told me to act.

Dear Shela:
It is being very hard for me to accept my memory loss. I know now that I do have one and am sometimes unable to recognize even my wife and my

children. It hurt me to find that I could not call you by name while I was a guest in your home. Please forgive me for the many times I thought you were someone else. I was merely seeing and saying what my mind told me to say and to see.

THIRD AND FINAL STAGE

The patient moves from the first stage of personality changes due to short-term memory loss on into the turbulent second stage filled with agitation, confusion, and disorientation caused by increased memory loss. In the final stage, according to Nancy L. Mace and Peter V. Rabins, "so much of the nervous system is failing that the rest of the body is profoundly affected." Patients in the final stage often have to be fed and toileted, as they may now be completely incontinent and sometimes even unable to walk or talk. As Barry Reisberg states, "The brain appears to no longer be able to tell the body what to do."[17]

Since Hughes is still in the late second or perhaps early third stage, I asked a caregiver who has had experience with the final stage to give her account of its symptoms. I first met Jean—a widow with grown children who works part time—in 1988 when I took Hughes to the same day-care center that Jean's mother, Blanche, was attending. Blanche Mae Squier Woodruff, who died of Alzheimer's disease in 1990, was born in 1904 in Loup City, Nebraska. Jean took care of Blanche in the second and final stages of the disease, and I saw her in a "place" of acceptance and tenderness with her mother that was not yet a reality for me with Hughes.[18]

When Blanche was seventy-six years old, although she had spent most of her life as a homemaker, cooking and taking care of her family, home, and garden, she could no longer remember how to make a cake. Or she would take three different packages of meat from the freezer and forget to use them. Looking back, Jean feels that her mother might have been in the beginning stage of AD as early as age sixty-six: Jean recalls that when she moved into her own new home in 1970, Blanche never learned how to find her way to the bathroom there, even though the house was not large or complex. Her mother once said that if she did not come back from the bathroom, Jean should come and get her.

In 1984 Blanche's husband, Rollie, died. Prior to his own illness, Rollie had taken care of Blanche. On the day of his death, Jean moved into her mother's home, for Blanche by then needed twenty-four-hour care. In 1986 she was evaluated by a geriatric assessment clinic, which confirmed the diagnosis of AD. Before the onset of the disease, Jean says, her mother was a loving, warm, thoughtful person who would never say an unkind word to anyone. Yet now she verbally abused her daughter, struck her on more than one occasion, and once chased her with an iron skillet. In 1987 Jean was so uncertain of her own safety that she bought a trailer and had it moved next to her mother's house as a place of respite and quick retreat. Also in 1987 Jean began taking her mother to an Alzheimer's day-care center two or three times each week. Blanche had become so argumentative and combative that Jean requested medication from Blanche's psychiatrist to calm her down. According to Jean, the drug Navane was effective.

To illustrate the tiers in the final stage, Jean used the change in her mother's ability to speak. At the beginning of the first tier her mother could still put some words together. In the second tier her words became fewer and fewer until, in the last tier, she could speak only one word as a response to a question. According to Reisberg, some patients are able only to grunt in the end.

Jean outlined several additional symptoms displayed by her mother in the final stage.

REFUSAL TO EAT

In the earlier stages, Blanche was hungry all the time and could never get enough to eat, yet her constant eating did not stop her weight loss. In the final stage, however, she refused to eat.

EMACIATION

Blanche weighed eighty-six to ninety pounds before her death. Her skin was tissue thin; just lifting her would tear it. Sometimes Jean walked backward, facing her mother, leading her by her fingertips in order to avoid touching her arms. Also, the shoulder strap in Jean's car hurt Blanche's skin, so using an old seatbelt, Jean had a lap belt made for her mother at a leather shop.

STIFFENING OF JOINTS

It became harder and harder for Blanche to walk, stand up, or sit down. Jean used a pillow to lift Blanche up when she had been lying down. She slept in the fetal position and could not fully straighten her back or her limbs. It was difficult for her to get in and out of the car. Once she was on the car seat, Jean would slide her into position on a soft mat.

When Blanche could no longer get in and out of the bathtub, Jean laid a forty-foot carpeted trail on which she walked Blanche daily from her home to the shower in Jean's trailer. After a few months, walking became too difficult for Blanche, and Jean took her by car to her trailer. As Blanche grew still more frail, Jean had a shower installed in her mother's home a few feet from her hospital bed.

INCONTINENCE

Blanche had been incontinent for at least two years before her death.

REPETITIVE MOVEMENTS

Before walking became so difficult for Blanche, she would walk in place, not moving from one spot. Sometimes she walked into a corner and, unable to turn herself around, kept on walking in place before calling for Jean's help. Even though she did not seem to know Jean was her daughter, she never forgot her name, the only name she remembered.

INCREASED INABILITY TO RECOGNIZE FAMILY

Blanche often thought Jean was her mother and that she herself was a young girl living at home with her parents. In the final stage she seldom recognized any members of her family.

REDUCED EXPRESSION OF ANGER

The only times Blanche got angry in the last stage were when Jean took her dentures out for brushing. She always insisted she did not have false teeth.

According to Jean, Blanche always took pride in keeping up her appearance. About three weeks before her death, Jean took her to the beauty shop to get a permanent. She fed Blanche cookies to help her remain in the chair while the beautician styled her hair.

Blanche attended day care up to the week before her death. Her lungs filled with a heavy fluid, and she died at home in Jean's arms on 6 September 1990. Watching Jean take care of her mother was like watching a rare work of art.

THREE
The Humanity of the Alzheimer's Patient

Blanche did not always know who Jean was, but Jean always remembered who Blanche was, and she treated her mother like a human being—as if her life had value.

There is no element more central or more necessary for excellent careproviding than the acceptance of the AD patient as a human being, yet this basic concept of the humanness of the patient is all too often overlooked. When we deny another's humanness, however, we deny the existence of that person's inner spirit or soul. One reason slavery endured for so long in America was that some proponents promoted the idea that the Africans had no souls. It is a dangerous and degenerate society that engages in the dehumanization of any segment of its population.

It is precisely because Hughes is a human being that I believed it possible to take care of him in our home. Dementia or disease cannot destroy anyone's essential humanness. Humanness is a gift of birth. It is intrinsic to our being, to the life that we are. Dementia is just one of the legions of manifestations of what it means to be human. As one author puts it, "A lethal disease in old age is not necessarily a tragic outcome, but an inherent part of the human condition."[1]

My dictionary defines "human" as "characteristic of or relating to man or woman in his or her essential nature; . . . susceptible to, representative of, or exemplifying the range of feelings, strengths, or weaknesses of which man or woman is capable." We mortals often fail to include our "weaknesses" in our definition of what it means to be human (unless, of course, we are looking for a way to excuse ourselves). Yet being human includes both sickness and wellness, good and evil, old and new, positive and negative, saint and sinner.

In our so-called civilized society, we as individuals often dehumanize persons we perceive to be different from ourselves; likewise, the ruling majority as a group dehumanizes large segments of the population who fail the test of "normality" as standardized by the powers in control. Also, as mortals, we have long sought to quantify life in order to justify ourselves and our actions. Thus, in any discussion of the humanity of the AD patient, one must acknowledge the ongoing and unresolved debate over "quality versus quantity" of life. But while ethicists, moralists, and religionists dispute among themselves, I believe the answer, like beauty, "is in the eye of the beholder."

An AD patient's care requires major life changes for the involved family members. It interferes with our plans for our own lives. Overnight, our world is turned upside down. It is little wonder that many of us prefer to think of AD as being outside the human experience. Such reasoning permits us to excuse ourselves from dealing with the patient or the disease. In other words, when they can no longer relate to the patient in the usual and customary way, some families and friends refuse to relate altogether. Some people act as if the AD patient were already dead. It is not unusual for the caregiver and the patient to be abandoned by family members and isolated by friends at a time when human contact with others is their greatest need.[2] The AD patient, especially in the beginning stage, needs continual interaction and human stimulation. But once a person is diagnosed with the disease, human contacts are often the first to go.

Family and friends often rally around when one has a physical illness, but it is quite a different story when a mental impairment is involved. It is safe to say that because of our lack of continued involvement with AD patients, our society does not yet know what may be possible in their care and management. Sharon, one of the "sisters," told me, "As human beings, we have evolved physically, but we are still in prehistoric times when it comes to our mental development."

A hundred or even fifty years ago, persons with manic depression and schizophrenia were for the most part simply shunned and locked up.[3] Today there are more treatment programs for them and also training and counseling programs for their families, enabling the mentally ill to live in varying degrees of independence in the community.[4] I do not believe the books have been written yet on what is possible for the physically healthy AD patient—one who is not given tranquilizing drugs and who is accepted and treated like a human being in the community of family and friends.

Facing the person who has AD means doing a new thing. It means taking a risk. Initially, it means feeling uncomfortable and uncertain. It requires a stretching of ourselves into dimensions of consciousness, growth, and pain that our minds could not have imagined. But for those of us who feel we must face and care for the person with AD, the first step is acceptance of the patient as another human being.

Although very little has been written on the humanness of persons who are cognitively impaired, two social scientists at Syracuse University, Robert Bogdan and Steven J. Taylor, conducted a four-year study on the social construction of humanness among severely disabled people, many of whom had been diagnosed as severely or profoundly retarded.[5] Many had an IQ (intelligence quotient) below twenty, some so low that they were considered untestable. Bogdan and Taylor state, "We argue . . . that the definition of a person is to be found in the relationship between the definer and the defined, not determined either by personal characteristics or the abstract meanings attached to the group of which the person is a part." The patients in the study sometimes "drooled, soiled themselves, and did not talk or walk—traits that most would consider highly undesirable," but their care-providers "accepted them as valued and loved human beings," recognizing "the severely disabled as 'someone like me,' that is, as having the essential qualities to be defined as a human being." Some caregivers "took the role of the other" and tried to "imagine what the patient would feel in the particular situation." They did not deny the disability, but they viewed it as secondary to the person's essential humanness. (As psychologist, Chris Milne, puts it, "Hughes is more than his memory.")

In contrast to "the dehumanizing perspectives often held by institutional staff and others in which people with severe disabilities are viewed as non-persons or subhuman," Bogdan and Taylor found, "the nondisabled care-givers [in the study] view the disabled people as full-fledged human beings." These caregivers demonstrated their perception of the humanness of their patients in *four* ways: they believed that the patients could think; they saw individuality in the patients; they thought of the patients as reciprocating; and they felt that the patients defined social place for them.

According to Bogdan and Taylor, the caregivers in their study "believe and cited evidence that their disabled partners [patients] can and do think. . . . Some people stated emphatically that they know exactly what the disabled person thinks. . . . With the limited range of gestures and sounds that many severely disabled people have, one might think such understanding would be extremely difficult. But these nondisabled people said this is not the case for them. . . . They said they can read gestures and decipher signs of the inner state of the other that strangers cannot see. For instance, some claimed that they can understand their partners by reading their eyes." The study tells of one three-year-old boy who was blind and completely paralyzed; he could only make slight movements with his tongue and a slow rolling of his eyes. The doctors and social workers told the foster parents that "he had no intelligence," but the caregivers maintained that observing the changes in the movement of his tongue and eyes indicated to them that he could "hear and recognize others."

Despite being "bombarded with specialists' judgments that, in their eyes, underestimate their partners' capabilities" caregivers argued that "specialists are not privy to the long day to day, hour by hour observation of the person. Behaviors that they cite as indicating understanding do not occur with such frequency that the professional is likely to see them. Further, unlike the nondisabled partners in these relationships, professionals are not intimately familiar with their clients and therefore are not attuned to the subtleties of their sounds and gestures." The caregivers in the study described the disabled persons as "distinct, unique individuals with particular and specific characteristics that set them apart from others." One foster father spoke of his daughter as "having a distinct personality, particular likes and dislikes, normal feelings and motives, a distinct background—in short a clear identity."

Bogdan and Taylor conclude: "Whether or not people with severe disabilities will be treated as human beings or persons is not a matter of their physical or mental condition. It is a matter of definition. We can show that they, and we, are human by including, by accepting them rather than separating them out.... What and who others, as well as we, are depends upon our relationships with them and what we choose to make of us."

With Hughes, I experience all the characteristics of humanness related by the caregivers in this study. Once he had come through the turbulent times of the second stage of AD, a calm seemed to come over him, and the distinctive qualities of his personality resurfaced: his personal charm, his willingness to share, his modesty, his concern for another's safety, and his display of affection. Of course, all his actions take place within the limitations of his remaining abilities to express himself. The results of his latest cognition test (1990) showed he had little to none. Yet despite all his deficits, when one engages Hughes, his humanness shines through his disease, and it becomes evident that he is indeed a distinct person and can still think. Throughout each day, his big wide eyes light up with life and laughter, with love and gratitude, and sometimes even mischief. He seldom shows or expresses any anger (one of his pre-AD characteristics). Once, however, when I scolded him, he told me, "Get out of my house!"

One activity he can still understand and enjoy is throwing a ball. Sometimes he pretends to throw the ball to you but, instead, throws it somewhere else and laughs, indicating he knows he has played a trick on you. He has a doll and a bunny he talks to, kisses, and hugs—much as he caressed our four babies. He places them on the couch next to him. When I try to sit on the couch, he frowns, protests, and rushes to scoop the doll and bunny up out of harm's way, making sure I do not sit on them.

On our walks he still jumps over mud puddles and walks around cracks in the sidewalk. If there is an obstruction in our path, he presses my hand to steer me away from what he perceives as danger. Two or three years ago, if we saw a small child alone on the street as we walked by, he would become very agitated, slowing down and looking back, pointing to the child. I am sure he thought the child was lost. Each time I had to reassure him that everything was all right before he would continue on our walk.

Hughes usually has to be directed how to wash his hands and what and where his towel is in order to dry himself. But before he will use the towel, he always examines it and avoids using the ends, thinking they may have been used before; he also smells his washcloth for freshness before using it—all pre-AD personal traits.

At meals he seldom eats without offering me some of his food, often the first bite. In his big family growing up, his mother had taught him that no matter how small the portion, it was always big enough to share. When he gets into his twin bed at night, often he positions his two pillows side by side beckoning to me to lie beside him.

When I scold Hughes, he frequently takes my hand and kisses it. His greatest show of affection is in the bathroom after I have settled him in for his toileting. He kisses my hand or cheek. It is as if he knows this is the most difficult part of his care, and this is his way of saying "thank you." Clearly, a loss of cognition is not a loss of one's feelings or one's humanity.

His response to another's show of affection for him is also predictably human. In the morning when our son Eric comes to take him to day care, he greets his dad with a hug and snuggling kisses. Before AD, Hughes was too macho to submit willingly to his sons' physical affection. Now he is more accepting; he smiles and obviously enjoys the touching and the attention. As our long-time friend Hugh Bullock said after observing Hughes's warm response to Eric, "Everybody knows love."

I believe I understand what he is trying to communicate to me 99 percent of the time, despite his unintelligible speech. Of course, this is partly due to our having lived together for forty-eight years, but more important, I respond instinctively to him as one human being to another. As many of the caregivers in the Bogdan and Taylor study said, "Intuition is the source of understanding people with severe disabilities and what they think. As the parent of a profoundly retarded young woman explained when asked how she knows what her daughter understands: 'It's just something inside me. . . . I really believe that deep in my soul.'" Many of the problems we face in patient care are solved when we remember the human factor.

For a better understanding of the humanness of AD patients, one need only compare their ability to feel with the ability of an infant to feel. We do not question that babies have feelings, despite their limited cognition, limited focus, and limited ability to communicate with us. We do not equate the babies' limitations with a lack of humanness. Why then would an AD patient, perhaps the grandfather or the grandmother of that baby, be less human?

We know that babies feel safe and secure and accepted when held by some people but threatened, unsafe, and unwanted when held by others. Babies know the presence of loved ones. It is the same with AD patients. As one wife puts it, when she visits her husband in the nursing home, "he doesn't know me, but he knows I belong to him."

I believe that Hughes, like other demented patients, is much closer to his feelings and basic instincts than so-called normal individuals, because in the process of becoming civilized and formally educated we often become separated from our feelings and skeptical of our instincts. We put our trust instead in written and visual information, purportedly proven by someone else. But when AD strikes, it is back to the basics. That is all the AD patient has left.

In fact, it appears that some of the patients' symptoms are responses to their situation deriving from basic instinct. Hughes's responses are typically human. As Shakespeare has Polonius say of Hamlet, "Though this be madness, yet there is method in it."[6] Take, for instance, the symptom of wandering. Eric says, "It's wandering to us, but it's probably for the most part going home to them."[7]

With little or no memory, the AD patient feels lost, confused, and disoriented. Nothing looks familiar. The patient begins desperately searching, trying to find something, someone, anything recognizable. Perhaps it was AD that made Shakespeare's King Lear ask,

> Does any here know me? This is not Lear.
> Does Lear walk thus? speak thus? Where are his eyes?
> Either his notion weakens, or his discernings
> Are lethargied—Ha! waking? 'Tis not so.
> Who is it that can tell me who I am?[8]

One can hardly imagine the fears that surely beset the AD patient. In the beginning stage, Hughes acted as if he had lost something and could not find it. Anyone who is lost instinctively tries to find the way back home— hence the wandering. The loving caregiver continually provides reassurance that the patient is loved and safe and will be all right, hoping that "Home is where the heart is" will become a reality for the AD patient through constant reassurance and loving care.

The "method in the madness" of hiding possessions is also logical and human. We so-called normal individuals often assume that the person with whom we live has mislaid our possessions when we cannot find them. How many of us have called out to a spouse, "Honey, did you pick up my glasses" or "Have you put my socks somewhere?" Since AD patients can no longer recognize objects, they cannot "find" them. When the careprovider "finds" them, patients then hide their possessions to make sure that no one can take them away again.

The symptom of spontaneous weeping is also a logical response to the patients' sense of personal loss. I believe that when Hughes wept, he was mourning that part of himself he was losing. In the first tier of the beginning stage, I do not believe he knew consciously what was happening to him. But when he progressed to the second tier of the first stage, he knew. In 1986 he wondered aloud if he had "that Alzheimer's disease" and requested me to make a doctor's appointment for him. Spontaneous weeping provides a safe release valve for patients at a time when they still have some fleeting understanding that a dreadful disease has seized them and is beyond their control.

The humanness of Hughes is also evidenced in remnants of ego and vanity. He may not open his mouth for me to start brushing his teeth, but he always cooperates after I whisper in his ear, "You have bad breath." In the words of the Preacher in Ecclesiastes, "All is vanity"—even in dementia. Hughes's ego still responds to challenges to his abilities, however faint the response. He tries harder to perform when asked, "Do you know how to stand on your feet, or how to get in the car, or how to sit on the toilet seat?" (Patients may forget how to do everything.) Confronting him with "Do you know" apparently triggers his ego to call upon all his remaining resources.

Fortunately, the "personhood" concept of demented individuals is slowly being advocated and manifested in a growing number of nursing facilities in the United States and other countries as they change from a "medical model" to a "social model" (see chapter 10). Concurrently, however, there are others who question whether people with AD are still "persons." Indeed, some presume to define who qualifies to be a person, and some argue that the money spent on AD patients is a "waste."[9] But the meaning of "waste" is defined by our values, and values and "waste" are determined individually.

In 1991 Americans spent $258.7 billion on personal consumption for recreation.[10] Was that a "waste"? It was almost four times the costs of AD care for that year. David H. Smith states: "Our images of the demented as sources of shame, or as beings who suffer in isolation, or as people who can be discounted reflect our images of ourselves. They show us the strengths and limits of what we value about our lives. I think we should recognize the dignity of the demented as part of our lives and the lives of those we love, and as refracted images of ourselves."[11]

Each of us has our task and mission in life until we complete our life cycle. Hughes has had many missions throughout his lifetime (demonstrated by the examples of his writings in the appendix). It is his nature to fulfill his task to the maximum. He was a revolutionary, always on the front line, standing up for the human dignity of any individual or group of individuals being treated as less than human. He was representing the civil rights of women and religious minorities through his government union long before they were popular causes.[12] Also, I remember how shocked some of our children were in the early 1980s to read in the newspaper that their father had been one of the main speakers at the first rally held in Lincoln to support human rights for persons with a gay or lesbian life-style. But he felt strongly the humanness of all people.

I see Hughes today as still contributing. His task at this time is to be an AD patient. I do not try to shield or protect Hughes from living with the consequences of AD. That is why I choose not to give him any drugs that would function to deny him the reality of his condition, however modified that reality may be. He appears to have no pain and seems content. He requires no pity, only respect. He is fulfilling his mission by prompting others to examine current attitudes and policies on what is possible in the care and management of Alzheimer's patients. It is through the profundity of his humanness that he is training me. I believe he knows somewhere inside that he is still fighting for the human dignity of the individual. Every AD patient offers us an extraordinary opportunity to discover more enlightened approaches to patient care and to advance the human race to new frontiers of understanding.

Once when Hughes was confused and would not cooperate and I was so angry, I prayed, "God, let me see You in Hughes even when he seems so ugly and unlovable." The answer came back swift and clear: "When you see Me in you—then you will see Me in Hughes."

It is in the engagement of other human beings that we are able to experience their humanness and the fulfillment of our own.

PART TWO
Techniques for Successful In-Home Management

FOUR
Learning to Live in the World of Dementia

Immediately after Hughes's AD was diagnosed, I began preparing myself mentally for a long undertaking. I remembered his mother, Susan, who lived to be ninety-seven; for twenty or more years before her death in 1988 she had not been able to recognize Hughes or remember that he was her son. Like Hughes she had a strong body, but mentally she was incapable of living alone and taking care of herself. She was never diagnosed as having a dementia, however; her doctor simply called it "senility." Hughes's father, Charles, died at age sixty-five of complications from a blood clot.

Just as the life expectancy of one diagnosed with AD varies from person to person, so does the rate of progression of the disease.[1] The fifty-one-year-old woman who was first diagnosed by Alois Alzheimer in Germany in 1906 as having this strange new disease died four and one-half years later. Dr. Alzheimer said of her that "mental regression advanced quite steadily."[2] Some AD patients, however, live ten, twenty, or more years with the disease.[3]

In preparation for a possible long stint in caring for Hughes, I began researching and reading every book and article I could find on the disease. I knew I needed to know as much as possible about AD. I also needed a plan, a strategy for how I would proceed to take care of Hughes.[4] At the same time I needed a plan for living out my own life to the fullest. After thirty-five years I was finally free of parental responsibility, and I had looked forward to the day when our children were all grown and independent. And now that I was retired, I had entered a wonderful new stage in my own personal development. At last I could do some of the things I had waited to do all my life. Hughes's diagnosis did not change that. I was more determined than ever.

As I began my research on AD, I felt certain there would be information that would help me develop a plan for his care. Yet everything I read about the families affected by AD was filled with hopelessness and despair. Even the titles of the books were depressing, and they all began and ended with the same theme: "Caregivers, prepare yourselves to live a life straight out of hell."

But given my heritage, the experience of hell on earth was not new to me. I had found that facing each new difficulty always gave me new inner strength. I had watched my mother confront adversity head-on: the more difficult the task, the more determined she became. I could do no less. She always said each generation should be an improvement over the last generation.

I had also learned over a lifetime not to make difficult experiences the whole of my life. I felt that Hughes's illness had a larger meaning and purpose beyond his loss or my loss. Even in the beginning stage when I was so enraged and resentful, feeling all alone, not knowing what to do next, I still knew within that there were logical, humane, and intelligent solutions to every problem I faced with Hughes. But I had to get beyond my rage and self-pity before I could see them.

I began contemplating Hughes's having AD from the broadest possible world view I could muster. From that perspective, I told myself to think of our home as a laboratory where my job was to observe both Hughes and me; from my observations I would learn what to do. I knew I had to be as detached, impersonal, and objective as possible, but it was hard to be objective in those early days. Every minute with Hughes was a challenge.

In 1995 I found in Hughes's desk a note that he had probably written many years before in the beginning stage of his disease:

> Hughes H. Shanks
> Steps you need to take:
>
> 1. Take clothes off.
> 2. Take bath or wash up.
> 3. Put on pajamas.
> 4. Say prayers.
> 5. Go to bed.

Over the years I have seen him struggling, always trying to connect, grasping to hang on to bits and pieces of what little of his previous reality he had left. When he began to hide his possessions, behavior that seemed bizarre to others reflected his best efforts to survive. Slowly, I began to help him with tasks. At bedtime, when it took him longer and longer to figure out how to get his clothes off and get ready for bed, he gradually permitted me to take on more and more of his personal care. It was then that I realized Hughes was beginning to adapt and learn how to live in his new world of dementia.

Although I knew that we humans are the most adaptable of all creatures, could this be true of an AD patient? I thought of Darwin's theory of the survival of the fittest. If, indeed, it is true, could it be applicable to an AD patient? I did not find any such references or ideas in the books and articles I read. I needed some validation of what I thought was happening.

I also observed that Hughes was progressing more rapidly in the disease—although he still had periods of lucidity—than I was learning or changing. I was stumbling upon some solutions to the problems presented by his new behavior, but I was floundering and knew I needed help. I felt overwhelmed, and I still had no clear plan or sense of direction for managing Hughes in our home. Yet I knew there must be a way to understand his behavior and a way to establish a new sense of normality in our lives. But to whom would I turn?

In 1988 Eric and I started attending meetings of the local Alzheimer's Association support group for the families of patients. We knew some of the members, and we were warmly welcomed and embraced by everyone. I quickly found out I was not alone. It was comforting to meet people who understood what I was going through. I felt a real camaraderie. Many of the members reminded me of veterans who had survived a long and brutal war and could not stop talking about it. In the beginning the meetings were invaluable, providing an outlet for all my negative feelings. Gradually, however, I wanted to go beyond the negativity and move to a discussion of positive solutions. I knew that in order to go on with my life and live it as completely as possible, I had to find a way beyond the pain and suffering. I had to learn to make the pain work for me.

I thought of the Veterans Administration. Hughes had always had a great respect for the VA. It was the VA that interceded on his behalf in the 1950s when no federal agency would hire him, despite his law degree and qualifying scores that placed him at the top of the registers of several federal agencies. Hughes had seldom turned to the VA for medical assistance, even though he had a service-connected disability; he had felt that it was his responsibility to pay for his own care. But now perhaps it was time to ask the VA for help. I knew that veterans' services were being cut, but given his war injury, maybe Hughes would be eligible for help. I made an appointment with the local Veterans Administration Medical Center. In our first interview, I was told he could not qualify to see a psychiatrist on a regular basis, but because of his Purple Heart he was eligible to visit a psychologist. Initially, however, a psychiatrist interviewed Hughes and suggested that I put him in the VA hospital for a week so that they could test him further. I respectfully declined; Hughes had already been tested twice. More important, I knew how confused and agitated he became in a new and strange environment, and I did not want to risk his disorientation or his being sedated or given some mind-altering drug. Instead, I was thankful to make an appointment to see a psychologist.

AN AD PATIENT CAN STILL LEARN

We were assigned to Chris Milne, Ph.D., in the VA's mental health clinic. When I first saw Dr. Milne, my heart sank. He looked so young, younger than Eric! Oblivious to my own ageism, I thought, "What a young whippersnapper! What does he know that can help us?" To my great surprise and excitement, by our second visit Dr. Milne was giving me the information I needed to begin our plan for survival. He told me that people who were demented could still learn![5] I thought, what a miracle! It wasn't just wishful thinking or a pipe dream after all, this idea of successfully taking care of Hughes at home. Despite AD, Hughes could still learn! Dr. Milne made it clear that it was not easy for a demented person to learn, but that given repetition, over and over again, it was possible.

Dr. Milne asked what in Hughes's behavior currently caused me the greatest stress. That was easy: his hiding of personal items he needed to use daily—his razor, toothbrush, eyeglasses, hairbrush, and others. Dr. Milne told me to take charge of his personal things and, every time I handed Hughes an object such as his toothbrush, to tell him to be sure and return it to me. It worked! In the beginning, I hung around while he brushed his teeth to remind him. I used this procedure with every toilet article I gave him. Eventually, it became automatic for him to return everything he had in his hands to me. If he picked up a chair or even a piece of paper, he would bring it to me. Sometimes he referred to me as the boss, saying he had to return this or that item to the boss. He still had periods of some lucidity, but more and more often he did not know who I was.

Nevertheless, the knowledge that an AD patient could still learn opened up a whole new world of possibilities for me as I worked with Hughes. It provided the foundation for managing him in our home. Rather than thinking that Hughes could not do something, after visiting with Dr. Milne I began to think that maybe he could—not in the old way, of course, but in some simple, basic, modified fashion (realistic expectations are essential for successful AD patient management). This attitude led me to discover that I could "trigger" a desired response from Hughes. I learned that the body remembers what the mind forgets. Much of our behavior is reflexive; for instance, when we brush our teeth, we don't have to think about it to do it. Likewise with Hughes—but in order to trigger that action in him, I had to start brushing his teeth and then put his left hand on the toothbrush handle as it was moving. It appeared that the back-and-forth motion of the brush in his mouth prompted something in him to take over this once familiar activity.

Hughes has now progressed so far in the disease that he has forgotten how to initiate any of the actions necessary for his personal care. As late as 1993, however, when I took the time to use the triggering method, in addition to brushing his teeth he could perform several functions for himself: wash his face and hands; dry his hands; put on his socks and shoes; tie his shoes; blow his nose; wipe his mouth; and feed himself. In each of these activities the triggering principle seemed to kick in when I properly positioned his hands or feet in relation to his body or the objects involved: that is, I tried to mimic as closely as possible the way Hughes performed these actions for himself before AD. Example: Hughes always put his socks and shoes on with one leg crossed. Thus, I would cross his leg and place his hands on the sock I had started putting on his foot. Something clicked then, and he took over. According to Dr. Milne, the more he repeated an action, the more it became reinforced in him, despite the AD.

Basic to assisting him in performing any function is an awareness that he is left-handed. It is so important when working with an AD patient not to take anything for granted, remembering the humanness and individuality of the patient. I believe that even without any training, an accepting caregiver who is not blinded by anger and rage eventually learns intuitively the necessary techniques for good patient care.

Dr. Milne validated my belief that it was possible to manage an AD patient in the home successfully for an extended period of years without the use of sedating or tranquilizing drugs.

AN AD PATIENT NEEDS STRUCTURE

The second most important lesson I learned from Dr. Milne was that the AD patient would function best in a structured environment. Gradually, I began to alter and adjust the physical features of our home to meet Hughes's changing needs.

BATHROOM CHANGES

When I awakened one morning at three o'clock and found Hughes in the bathtub, singing and running water full blast as he took his third bath that night, I called our friend Dean Achen to put shutoff valves on the bathtub faucets. Hughes no longer had an awareness of night and day. His sense of time was gone.

He also went through a period of removing all the clean towels, washcloths, and toiletries from the bathroom, hiding them in his favorite places. When I was still in some denial that he had AD, I tried unsuccessfully to reason with him. Eventually, I stripped our bathroom of all linens except the towels on his rack, all toiletries, and all cleaning agents, since by then he would drink any liquid. I made a place for myself in our upstairs bathroom.

At the time Hughes mistook the furnace floor vent for a bathroom urinal, I remember feeling so distressed; it seemed the biggest problem I had faced yet. Fortunately, the incident happened in the summer when the furnace was off. I first consulted with several furnace companies as to whether I could move the vent from the floor to the wall—but I was not sure Hughes would not use a wall vent as well. After meditation, it came to me simply to place a cookie sheet over the opening. I had one already on hand that completely covered the vent, and I never had that problem again. Then, when Hughes confused the washbasin and bathtub with the commode, I consulted with our son Cedric on one of his visits. He constructed three partitions out of wall paneling, held together by hooks, which hid the basin and tub from Hughes; the only opening left was the commode. Later our friend Neil reinforced the partitions to make them stronger. The paneling is very light, and I put the three pieces in place every night.

BEDROOM CHANGES

The most painful structural change was to separate our twin beds and move mine to another room. In retrospect, however, I know it was one of the wisest changes I made (see the discussion of emotional detachment in chapter 8).

By 1988 Hughes more and more frequently did not know who I was, and I never knew from minute to minute what he might do next. One morning I was startled when I opened my eyes to see him staring over at me, pointedly quizzing, "Who are you?" I thought it best to get right out of bed, all the while trying to explain, "I am Lela, your wife." In those days, when he still frequently thought I was an impostor trying to break up his marriage, there were times when I was not sure about my own safety. It seemed sensible for me to begin sleeping in another room where I would feel safer.

By the time I began disassembling my bed, however, Hughes was back to lucidity. He could not figure out why I was doing this. He was terribly hurt, and I could not make him understand. I kept quiet as I worked, moving furniture from room to room. He just stood there in the middle of divided mattresses and sheets, looking forlorn and helpless, asking why I was moving out and what he had done wrong. But AD can also be merciful. Hughes did not retain enough of the incident even on that day to come back to it—though for many nights afterward when he got into bed he always moved to one side, expecting me to lie down beside him.

After I moved into the back room, Hughes began urinating in his walk-in closet. He was also going through the phase of dressing and redressing. At this point I realized it was time to take charge of his clothing. On one of Cedric's visits, I moved all Hughes's clothes to a basement closet and Cedric nailed his closet shut for the duration.

I have been asked how I could just nail a closet shut. My answer is, how could I not nail his closet shut? How could the use of a closet compare to doing what is necessary to keep Hughes in his own home? Our daughter-in-law Chris observed that when a family member has a physical illness, we think nothing of making the structural changes necessary to facilitate home care. But not so with family members who have what we call mental illnesses (as if mental illnesses have no connection to the body). Nothing material compares to the value of a human life.

GATES AND LOCKS

After the incident when Hughes wandered off in 1991, I went to a lumberyard and discussed with a salesman the materials needed to install permanent gates and locks for the front porch, and also for Hughes's bedroom and bathroom entrances. A neighbor next door agreed to do the work, and within three or four days he had put a patio lock on our front porch door and installed four-foot-high plywood gates with patio locks on Hughes's bedroom and bathroom doors. Since the two rooms adjoin, this gives him a large safe secure area to use when necessary. I also had an electronic security system installed. When the alarm is set and Hughes opens the front or back door, the alarm alerts me.

COMPETENCY THEORY

As Hughes has progressed through the first two stages of the disease, I have seen him adapt to a new level of functioning in each tier. Of course, each new level is lower than the last; still, he reaches a plateau of adaptation on each tier and maintains it until more deterioration sets in.[6] I believe that from the onset of the disease, in the midst of all the confusion, the patient him- or herself is trying to establish some pattern for living in this unfamiliar environment.

I further believe that in an atmosphere of acceptance and in an AD-structured environment, it is possible for a patient to reach some level of competency for living in this strange new world of dementia.

FIVE
The Alzheimer's Patient and Cleanliness

In America's materialistic and youth-oriented culture, it is not unusual to find a subtle and sometimes outright contempt for older people.[1] With sky-rocketing health-care costs, some taxpayers agree with the former governor of Colorado, Richard D. Lamm, that when we reach our late seventies or early eighties "medical care should only be provided to relieve suffering."[2] Others predict an intergenerational war as the fight heats up over entitlements. Definitely, old is not in.

In our disposable society we throw away what we do not need anymore. Old people are burdens. Old means less valuable, less deserving. Old is unattractive. Old is nonproductive. The writer Margaret Walker, in her poem "For My People," calls for "a world that will hold all the people . . . and their countless generations."[3] But in America we have not yet discovered that our country is big enough to hold all the people. The worth of the individual is all too often determined by occupation, income, and age. No one wants to grow old.

It is out of this contempt for old people, along with a lack of information, that stereotypes and assumptions are born relating to their personal habits and living conditions. One assumption is that the elderly, demented or not, will naturally be less clean than the younger population; society's standards and expectations of cleanliness for them are therefore lowered. Comedians tell jokes about the "funny" smell of old people. Some older people themselves buy into this supposition, and it becomes a self-fulfilling prophecy.[4] It is generally when AD patients become incontinent and unable to attend to their own personal hygienic needs that our standards of cleanliness for them hit rock bottom. In fact, some families allow an elderly relative to live in unsanitary conditions that they would not tolerate for themselves, and some institutional care is no better.

INSTITUTIONAL LAPSES

The neglect of the elderly in regard to cleanliness and sanitation in many nursing homes has been well documented by the federal government. The Health Care Financing Administration (HCFA) keeps an ongoing record for all nursing homes in the United States of violations of the 264 federal regulations for long-term care facilities. (It is important to point out that these regulations were written to govern the medical model in nursing homes, not the social model or the AD special-care units discussed in chapter 10. In fact, however, some states are reinterpreting the regulations to cover the special-care units, which could positively affect the future care of AD patients in nursing homes.) The computerized HCFA tabulations are printed out, on request, in a document called "On-line Survey Certification and Reporting," or OSCAR. (Caregivers interested in getting a copy of the federal regulations or a printout of the OSCAR report should inquire at the offices of their state's health department.)

The record indicates that high percentages of the violations in nursing homes nationwide involve some aspect of sanitation and cleanliness. A total of 16,420 facilities were surveyed in OSCAR Report 18 (6 January 1994): 11,641 skilled nursing facilities (SNF), and 4,779 nursing facilities (NF). These are the two classifications of nursing homes as defined by HCFA; each state also has its own definition of SNF and NF (this information too may be obtained from the state department of health). Generally, however, patients in SNF require more care than do patients in NF, and the number of registered nurses on duty may be higher in SNF.

According to OSCAR Report 18, the highest percentage of violations in both SNF and NF (31 and 30 percent respectively) was the failure "to store, prepare, distribute, [and] serve food under sanitary conditions." The report further showed that five more of the ten regulations most frequently violated in NF related to some aspect of cleanliness:

1. 23 percent—providing the "housekeeping and maintenance services necessary to maintain a sanitary, orderly, and comfortable interior";
2. 15 percent—establishing "an infection control program" whereby the facility "investigates, controls, and prevents infections";
3. 15 percent—caring for residents "in a manner and in an environment that maintains or enhances each resident's dignity or respect in full recognition of his or her individuality";
4. 15 percent—providing "a safe, clean, comfortable and homelike environment, allowing the resident to use his or her personal belongings to the extent possible";
5. 14 percent—ensuring "a safe, functional, sanitary, and comfortable environment for the residents, staff and the public."

In SNF, half of the top twenty regulations most frequently violated involved sanitation and cleanliness, nine in addition to the matter of sanitary food:

1. 21 percent—as in (3) above;
2. 18 percent—as in (4) above;
3. 15 percent—as in (2) above;
4. 13 percent—as in (1) above;
5. 12 percent—providing the care necessary to ensure that "a resident who is incontinent of bladder receives appropriate treatment and services to prevent urinary tract infections and to restore as much normal bladder function as possible";
6. 11 percent—caring for residents "in a manner and in an environment that promotes maintenance or enhancement of each resident's quality of life";
7. 10 percent—as in (5) above;
8. 10 percent—ensuring that "a resident having pressure sores receives necessary treatment and services to promote healing, prevent infection and prevent new sores from developing";
9. 9 percent—ensuring that "a resident who enters the facility without pressure sores does not develop pressure sores unless the individual's clinical condition demonstrates that they were unavoidable."

These are all matters that concern every caring family member who considers nursing home placement for a loved one. Without question, living conditions in American nursing homes for the elderly have been far worse in the past.[5] But as a country we still lack the moral will to treat old people as equal members of the human family. It is, therefore, up to the caregiver in the home and the chief executive officer (CEO) of the institution to set and maintain a high standard of cleanliness for the patient. Their attitudes will be the determining factors. When the CEO believes it possible and essential to maintain a clean, odor-free institution, this message is transmitted to each old and new employee through required, ongoing in-service training. If the boss feels that it is necessary and important for patients to wash their hands before meals, the staff will see to it that the patients' hands are washed.

HOME CARE AND CLEANLINESS

In the years Hughes has had AD, I have found it possible to keep a patient clean in body and in clothing. I have also found it possible to keep our home environment clean, sanitary, and entirely pleasant. This is one of the reasons I want to care for Hughes at home as long as I can. I want to maintain the same standard of dignity in his personal hygiene that he held for himself.

There are three necessary components in my program to keep Hughes clean:

1. the will to do so, coupled with the physical strength and physical mobility;
2. creative techniques for day-to-day problem solving, some derived from the suggestions of others, but most intuitive (the solutions often unfold and develop in the heat and midst of the problem);
3. an array of supplies, such as cleaning and sanitizing agents, incontinent briefs (diapers), bed protector pads, drawsheets, disposable washcloths, disposable gloves (no quantity of supplies, however, will help without the caregiver's will and determination).

The degree to which we identify with patients as fellow human beings largely dictates our attitude toward their cleanliness. As noted above, the prejudices of ageism can blot out the value of an old life. On the other hand, it is important to me as an individual to have a clean body, wear fresh clean clothes, and live in a clean, healthy, odor-free environment. I want the same for Hughes.

Once, Hughes became violently ill in the middle of the night. When I had put him to bed earlier, there was no warning or indication he was even feeling sick. In his present stage of the disease, he cannot verbalize how he feels. Sometimes he places his hands on his abdomen or his chest, indicating discomfort, but AD patients well into the second stage generally cannot tell us when they are in pain or where it hurts.[6]

Suddenly, I was awakened to find him dashing for the toilet. He did not make it, although he tried; bodily fluids were gushing and splattering in all directions. Momentarily, I could not move; I was overwhelmed, and for a brief second my mind could not accommodate the enormity of the cleanup. Where would I begin? I thought, "Now this is just why families put the patient in a nursing home." But as I stood there, frozen, I remembered similar incidents from years before when our four children had had upset stomachs and these same symptoms. I reminded myself that this was not a new experience. As a full-time homemaker I had spent a minimum of three years with each child (that is, twelve nonstop years) on the regurgitating and evacuation cleanup detail. I was a veteran at such cleanups. I also knew how to wipe and clean bottoms. I went into action, quickly grabbing newspapers, recalling how they can be used strategically for damage control.

After cleaning out a path, the first and most important thing to do was to clean and comfort Hughes. Suddenly, I was thankful he was not in a nursing home. I wanted to get him clean, to make his environment spotless. I kicked my shoes off, put on my rubber gloves, and waded in. It did not seem wise to put Hughes in the bathtub, since he was continuing to eliminate. Instead, I washed him up, put two incontinent briefs on him, dressed him in clean pajamas, and put him back to bed. Next I began a complete cleanup. On my knees, mopping the floor, I began to sing, realizing this was nothing more than work. Afterward, I made newspaper paths from his bed to the toilet for Hughes to use until he was over his illness. I brought in deodorizers and electric fans to disperse the odor.

There never was a time when I questioned whether I should keep Hughes in our home. To do so was a part of my heritage, my culture—a natural decision, given our relationship and our long life together. At best, though, the job of keeping another human being's body clean is formidable, not a task for the fainthearted. Caregiving as such is a process—an evolutionary process, a learning process. Caregivers are learners first. We learn as we go along. I did not have to learn everything all at one time, because it was over a period of years that Hughes gradually became incapable of taking care of himself. But as his abilities declined, I eased into the responsibilities of attending to his hygienic needs.

UNDRESSING FOR THE BATH

At the outset, I realized it would be best to go with the flow of the patient's usual habits as much as possible. For example, Hughes had always hated showers but loved taking long warm baths. Every experienced caregiver I talked with and everything I read indicated that AD patients in general hated to bathe.[7] But I quickly discovered that it was not the bath Hughes hated; it was giving up his clothes, especially to a "stranger." Trying to undress him in those early months was like tangling with a semi-friendly bear.

At first he resisted all my efforts, however politely, to try to help him wash. Back then he was still talking, but he did not know who I was most of the time. When I knocked first and then went into the bathroom with him, he would say, "Are your folks at home? Do they know you are in here?" or "You shouldn't be in here," or "You had better get out of here or we are going to get into trouble." It was not simply as if he was returning to his childhood but as if the record of his memory was replaying backward in turn each of the stages of his life. At this point he seemed to have regressed to his teenage years. By accepting him as a teenager mentally, I was able to come up with creative strategies for taking over his personal care. Even though I was still in some denial, when I finally changed from saying angrily in exasperation, "Man, we aren't teenagers! I am your wife!" to "No, my parents aren't home. We have the house all to ourselves—" well, I gradually established the regimen necessary for washing and bathing him. Naomi Feil named this method of entering the person's inner world "validation therapy."[8]

One time in the early years, after I had struggled to get all his clothes off, he stood nude, sadly shaking his head: "Now, I don't have anything," he said. After that incident I stopped taking all his clothes off at one time. Instead, I led him to his usual place on the couch, where he is comfortable, and told him I was going to give him a massage. As I removed his shoes (putting them far out of his reach), I continued to reassure him as I gently caressed and stroked his feet. (Hughes had given me foot massages throughout our marriage, but this was the first time it had occurred to me to do the same for him.) After his massage, he was more willing to give up the next piece of clothing. On some cold winter days, I even begin his bath by washing his feet in warm water as he sits on the couch. He is visibly soothed and calmed by those foot baths.

Today he stands quietly, cooperating, while I clean his body. Sometimes he stares at me longingly with that old familiar look of love and says (hardly audibly), "Thank you."

VELCRO TAPE IN THE CLOTHING

Hughes was always prudish, and his most prized piece of clothing continues to be his pants. Even today, despite all his mental deterioration, he still understands enough to want to hang on to them. In the beginning, getting Hughes to take his pants off for a bath or to change clothes for bed was the most stressful part of his care. I knew there had to be a better way. I called Ron, his son, by his first marriage, who was an engineer and lived in New Jersey. I told him the problem. He knew that I made Hughes's pants, and I asked him to design a pants pattern for his father that would eliminate the problem. Ron immediately suggested inserting Velcro fastening down one side! That was the solution I needed!

At first, I did this to every garment in sight—pants, shorts, undershirts, outer shirts, pajama tops and bottoms—but I quickly learned I needed the hook-and-loop tape only down the right side of all trousers, shorts, and pajama bottoms (the right side because that side faces me when I am working with him in the bathroom). Putting it in a pair of long pants or pajama bottoms is a simple process that takes only about thirty minutes, much less for a pair of shorts. Using pinking shears, I start at the pants hem and cut along the middle of the side seam right on through the waistband (sometimes I rip out the stitches rather than cut the seam, but that is optional). I pin the length of Velcro tape in place and stitch it in, always making sure that the rougher piece is sewn to the backside of the open seam, away from Hughes's skin. A minimum of sewing is needed to repair the hem and waistband seams. Now, whenever Hughes resists removing his pants, I distract him while opening the Velcro fastening; the pants or shorts fall to the floor and are off before he knows it. I continue to reassure him with strokes and caresses.

Like a child, Hughes is also fearful of anything going over his head. Since Velcro tape is difficult to use in stretchy knit fabric, I eliminated undershirts long ago. Instead, since he feels cold in both summer and winter, I make sure he wears two layers of buttoned clothing on his upper body. I cut the tails off all his inner button-down-the-front shirts to facilitate easy access to cleaning his intimate parts. Caregivers must approach every problem believing there is a more efficient way and tap into their own infinite storehouse of unlimited creativity.

Now that I am more experienced, in the winter I can sometimes slip a turtleneck shirt and a buttonless sweater over his head (before AD, he loved the warmth of turtlenecks). Occasionally, he even helps. I always praise him when he accomplishes anything. I learned from Eric to say, "Good man! Good job!" (Hughes responds well to Eric, and I thought "good man" sounded like a "male thing.")

Many caregivers find sweatsuits the best year-round clothing for AD patients, but Hughes never liked sweatsuits. In college he stood out because he was the only male in sight wearing a tie and jacket. The first time I saw him (in 1946) I thought, "How odd. He must be one of those old men coming back from the war." (He was.) He never looked casual. In those days of legal segregation he believed he always had to dress like someone going for a job interview. Today, whenever possible I respect his preferences.

GIVING HUGHES A BATH

Before giving Hughes a bath, I always make sure the bathroom is warm, almost hot. He responds to warmth. Once his clothes are off, he soon understands that he is to step into the water in the bathtub. I have a bathing stool but seldom use it, since he is still quite agile and able to sit down in the tub. I put a full-length nonskid rubber mat in the tub for his safety, and

I also assist him getting in and out. Occasionally, he does not remember how to get in or how to sit down or how to get up and step over the side. When that happens I have to wait him out. Eventually, with or without coaxing, he understands what to do.

Early on, I learned to use two washcloths, one for each of us. He was free to use his as he wished. I make lots of suds with liquid soap (I stopped using bar soap when he started eating it). When I shampoo his hair, I first mix the shampoo in my hand with warm water before putting it on his head. I continue to warm the water in the tub throughout his bath. When I finish washing him, he often stretches out in the tub singing and relaxing as he did before AD. After a while I remove the plug, and when Hughes observes the water going out, he stuffs his washcloth in the drain. When I take the washcloth out, he plugs it up with his heel. I often have to be very creative to get him up and out of the tub. I sometimes try to cue him with candy while calling his name and coaxing him to get out. The most effective way is to turn off the water valves in the cabinet behind the tub and leave him alone for a few minutes. When he cannot get any more water out of the faucets, he gets out on his own as if it is the natural thing to do. I then wrap him in a large towel and dry him off.

If for any reason I am unable to give Hughes a bath when he needs one, there are two or three options available: the adult day-care center he attends offers that service for a fee to its clients; I could pay a sitter or a professional home health-care worker to take over; or I could apply for help with Hughes through my state department of social services under a program called "Medicaid Home and Community-Based Services Waivers for the Elderly" (see chapter 10).

THE BODY WASHUP

On the days I do not put Hughes in the bathtub, I give him a washup, or sponge bath. In some ways, a washup is more satisfactory than a bath for total cleanliness of the patient. It is harder to wash his intimate parts while he is sitting in the tub.

I begin the washup while he is on the toilet. I try to occupy his hands with a book "to read"; otherwise, he is like an octopus. As with his bath, I start with his face, neck, and ears. Next I wash and dry his underarms and apply deodorant. I then help him to stand up. He seldom appears to remember how to stand erect anymore. He often stands with his legs apart and knees bent, holding on to the sink like a baby afraid of falling. As he faces the mirror and the washbasin, he waves and talks to the man in the mirror. Once he looked at himself and asked queryingly, "Hugh, is that you?" Sometimes he points to me as he talks to the man. He stands cooperatively as I thoroughly suds down his thigh and groin area. Sometimes he is incontinent of bladder in the night, and I want to remove all residue of urine from his body. I make sure to wash under the fold of fat on his lower abdomen and also in the inner areas of his groin. Washing these two places is critical to keeping a patient odor free. Also, since many men of Hughes's generation were not circumcised, it is imperative to pull the foreskin back and wash under it to avoid infection. Next I wash his bottom and the backside of his thighs. When I am finished, I dry him off and apply cornstarch or baby powder and body lotion appropriately.

IMPORTANCE OF INTIMATE CLEANSING

One cannot stress too much the need to give the AD patient this kind of intimate care. Even a prolonged tub soaking is no guarantee that a patient's anal area will be clean, especially AD patients. Since their mental impairment can diminish their rectal control, the result is often the retention of small particles of fecal matter around the rectum. A lack of intimate care is neglect; it can lead to infection and also contributes to the overall unpleasantness one encounters upon opening the front door of some nursing homes.

One of my sitters, whom I will call Carrie, is a junior nursing student at the University of Nebraska. She told about a bed bath she once gave a female patient—a woman of sound mind, but bedridden—in a nursing home. As Carrie proceeded to clean the patient's private parts, the frail woman looked at her with gratitude and softly exclaimed: "Oh, thank you, thank you. No one has washed me there since I have been in here. It feels so good to be clean." According to Carrie, the woman had been in the nursing home several months. It is ironic that some caregivers use "respecting the patients' privacy" as a reason for not changing their dirty diapers and cleaning their genitalia.

It is necessary to examine frequently the body of AD patients who can no longer express how they feel or tell us when they are in pain. This is especially important once the patient begins to experience any degree of incontinence. Dried urine can cause a breakdown of the skin, making the patient susceptible to sores and infections. That is why a daily washup of the body including the genital area is imperative. It is also necessary to apply lotion to the patient's body, especially during winter months. My longtime friend Omell McMillan, a quintessential caregiver, gave me the tip of massaging Hughes's buttocks with alcohol to toughen it against sores. In her fifty years of nursing dozens of bed-confined patients, none ever developed bedsores.

Likewise, my friend Genie Logan took care of her paralyzed husband, Percy, for eighteen years in their home, and he never had a pressure sore.

The caregiver, whether lay or professional, who respects the human dignity of the patient and wants to keep him or her clean finds a way. The caregiver who is overmodest or has a weak stomach quickly outgrows it. Personal care of the patient gets easier and more matter-of-fact with experience. Our daughter Shela, who could throw up on cue as a child, once remarked that she had a weak stomach until she had four children. I was not modest, nor did I have a weak stomach, but I was never a little girl who wanted to grow up and become a nurse. In AD caregiving, however, one is compelled to grow and develop in areas far beyond one's natural inclinations. I marvel that we can learn and adapt to new ways even in our old age, given the will and determination.

CARE OF NAILS

Keeping fingernails and toenails clean and clipped is a necessary part of an AD patient's care. Long, dirty, curved nails are one more sign of patient neglect. I had to learn how to cut Hughes's nails so that I would not hurt him. In the beginning, he was afraid and only reluctantly cooperated. I try to clip them at least once a week. I cut them across and not too close to the ends of his fingers and toes. He has one ingrown toenail, which I have learned to soak in warm soapy water before clipping. He is now able to relax when I groom his nails. As an alternative, some caregivers leave the care of the patient's nails to a podiatrist.

CARE OF TEETH

At seventy-six, Hughes still has his own teeth. I help him brush his teeth at least twice each day, in the morning when he arises and at night before he goes to bed. Since he is no longer able to initiate any activity, I always use the technique of "triggering," described in the previous chapter. Once I get him started, I say, "You do it. No one can brush your teeth as clean as you can." I constantly praise him. Once he gets started, I have to finally take the brush away from him. Often, he does not remember how to spit, but he has learned to accept water from my hand to rinse his mouth out. (When we take outside walks, however, Hughes always knows how to expectorate and does so several times, as if it is an automatic response. He is like a little boy who has just learned.)

Every year since he has had AD our dentist has cleaned his teeth. This has been a learning experience both for me and for the dentist. When Hughes reached the stage of not knowing either of us or what was going on, he resisted reclining in the chair. But our dentist was patient with him and persevered. For the past two or three years it has not been easy, but the dentist has continued to do what he can. He says we will take it one year at a time. Of course, trips to the dentist are stressful even for so-called normal people. Here again, Hughes adapted to what was necessary for living in the new world of dementia, and he has no cavities.

For the AD patient who wears dentures, the caregiver must remove and clean them every day. Jean Evans, who cared for her mother through the final stage of AD (see chapter 2), said that her dentist taught her how to get Blanche's teeth out by breaking the seal under the dental plate in her mother's mouth. She also told me that it is important to watch for sores under the plate, since the patient is often unable to verbalize any such problem.

CARE OF HAIR

I continue to take Hughes to the same barber who has cut his hair for the past thirty years. I try to take him every two weeks, keeping the same schedule he had before AD. At first, I felt a little awkward in a traditionally all-male barber shop, but I could not let that stop me. After several months I decided to have his barber cut my hair also. Hughes does not often understand immediately how to get into or out of the chair, but everyone is always patient and polite. In fact, our barber has offered to come to our home if Hughes becomes unable to go to his shop.

SHAVING

About four years ago, Hughes started leaving one side of his face unshaved. I could not get him to understand about the other half. For several months before that, I had assembled what he needed for shaving and used "triggering" to get him started. But one day he could not remember how to hold the razor anymore. Day after day, I tried to get him started with no success. He just stared at me blankly. It is helpful to remember that a one-time refusal to perform a task is not always a precedent; an AD patient will forget one minute and remember the next. And of course these fluctuations are an emotional roller-coaster ride for the caregiver. After several unsuccessful trials, however, I accepted that shaving was probably lost to Hughes forever.

But I had never shaved anyone before. Would I cut him? How much pressure is enough? He used a safety razor. He had tried different brands of electric razors many times but found them unsuitable for his curly hair.

I tried to visualize Hughes shaving as I had seen him countless times. He always said shaving day after day was terrible punishment to a man's face, but he was a creature of his time and shaved every day. I remembered his speaking of the need to keep one's razor clean and to use an astringent after each shave to avoid infection. He also kept a topical antibacterial ointment on hand for cuts.

I sought advice from our sons. They reminded me to put a warm, wet washcloth on his face before starting in order to soften his whiskers. I learned to be careful around his mouth, since he reaches with his lips for the razor. Today it takes about five minutes to give Hughes a shave. He is often amorous at this time, perhaps because of the proximity of our faces.

MANAGEMENT OF THE PATIENT'S CLOTHING

When Hughes began to put on two and three layers of clothing at one time, I realized that he was incompetent to make decisions about what to wear, even though he could still dress himself and still had brief periods of lucidity. I knew he needed help in the management of his clothes from day to day, and I decided to gradually start removing his clothes from his closet (this was before it became necessary to nail it shut). In the beginning he did not seem to notice, but as his closet emptied, he despaired, "Well, they are at it again. Somebody is stealing my clothes." I tried to reassure him by saying, "Oh, your clothes are at the cleaners," or "Your clothes are in the wash." Then I would distract him by talking about something else, and soon the clothes were forgotten. It never occurred to Hughes to look elsewhere in the house for them. Eventually, I kept two sets of clean clothing in his closet each day, giving him a choice as long as he could make a decision. But as he progressed in the disease he could not distinguish one piece of clothing from another. For a long time he could put on each item of clothing if I gave it to him along with assistance. But one day he could no longer remember what to do even with assistance, and I took over the total responsibility of dressing and undressing him.

When AD patients can no longer dress themselves, it is frequently the minutiae of activities for daily living (ADLs) that finally exhaust the caregiver and lead to the placement of the person in a nursing home. Little tasks like struggling to pull on tight socks every day take their toll: in one year alone the caregiver puts on or takes off a sock and shoe for the patient a minimum of 1,460 times. I put myself through months of unnecessary agony before it dawned on me to buy the most stretchable socks available. I quickly learned that one cannot rely on advertisements for stretch socks, since some have much less elasticity in the top and body than others. But I kept searching, and the socks I buy now are so stretchable they almost slide on by themselves.

I avoid tie shoes except for the days I take Hughes for walks. Instead, he wears a hard-soled house slipper called "Romeo," which are familiar to him because he wore them before AD.

ADULT INCONTINENT BRIEFS

When the AD patient begins to lose bladder or bowel control, protective briefs become a standard item of his or her clothing. There are several different styles for varying degrees of adult incontinence, and separate designs for men and women. At first, though Hughes seemed to have only a small leakage (I go into greater detail about incontinence in chapter 7), I searched every medical supply store in town and found styles ranging from knitted shorts with a panel in the crotch for holding a disposable pad to actual adult-size diapers. I bought two different styles of the knitted shorts and immediately put Velcro tape down one side, but I quickly found out these would not work with Hughes: at day care he sometimes came out of the bathroom with the pad in his back pocket. Next I tried an "undergarment" held on with a belt. Hughes took that off too. Meanwhile, he continued to lose bladder control, and in 1992 I reluctantly made the decision to begin using contoured incontinent briefs—adult diapers—on Hughes. Oh, how I dreaded it! But to my great surprise, Hughes immediately accepted wearing the new briefs. The truth is, he seemed relieved, despite my uncertainty and awkwardness at putting the first few on him. I thought, "How in the world do you put a diaper on a 175-pound moving man?" The first time, I backed him into a corner and somehow got it on. Then one of Hughes's old friends advised me to have him sit down. He was right, and after trial and error I found it best to put them on while Hughes is seated on the toilet. Today it is a snap. Hughes's quick acceptance and his adaptation to the bulky briefs is another example of his learning to live in his new world of dementia.

HAND WASHING

As patients progress in the disease, they often forget when or even how to wash their hands. They may not recognize the bathroom or a bar of soap, a washcloth, a towel, the water, or the washbasin. In the HCFA regulations on which the OSCAR reports are based, patient handwashing is not specified, but there is a regulation for staff handwashing, under "infection control": "The facility must require staff to wash their hands after each direct resident contact for which handwashing is indicated by accepted professional practice." According to OSCAR Report 18, staff handwashing violations were low nationally (6 percent for skilled nursing facilities and 5 percent for nursing facilities), though for my state they were high in NF, 22 percent, and 11 percent even in SNF.

But it is equally important to keep the patient's hands clean. Like a small child, Hughes will put his hands on anything anywhere. Before he sits on the toilet, he often touches the seat to assure himself he is not going to fall, because AD distorts his depth perception and impairs his judgment. Since he cannot recognize objects, he will pick up anything he sees on the floor or in the street. Receptacles are also very inviting to some AD patients. When I visited nursing homes after Hughes's diagnoses (see chapter 8), I shuddered to see patients rummaging through wastebaskets. Today, if a wastebasket is within Hughes's reach, he is like a scavenger.

I wash his hands frequently with warm water and soap and *always* after he uses the toilet, before he eats anything, and before he touches his toothbrush.

In sum, the test that I use for Hughes's cleanliness is the same standard that I hold for myself.

SIX
The Importance of Establishing Procedures

One statement made to me at the time of Hughes's diagnosis was that we could never live a normal life again. When I heard that, my first thought was, "The social worker does not know what she is talking about because there must be some normality in my life in order for me to be able to keep going day in and day out." Establishing detailed procedures for the total care of Hughes has helped to give our lives that normality and stability. I believe a regular routine has greatly facilitated his transition from living in a world of total confusion and disorientation to living in the new world of dementia. Thus, creating a structured environment for Hughes has benefited both of us.

As human beings we usually want and need a physical environment and an emotional climate that we can depend on—one in which we feel safe and secure.[1] An AD patient's loss of memory, followed by disorder and confusion, make structure and established procedures essential, especially in the earlier stages. I hasten to add, however, that rules for the activities of daily living (ADLs) cannot be set in stone; the caregiver has to be flexible, willing to change procedures that no longer work. Also, because each of us is an individual, caregivers will not all want the same kind or amount of structure. In fact, some may prefer not to have any structure at all, and some nursing homes use very little (see chapter 10). But for Hughes and me, structure and routine procedures have helped us to survive. It has also been helpful for me to write out detailed and up-to-date procedures on his care in order to ensure continuity whenever I must be absent.

Timing can often be everything in the care of the AD patient. The caregiver must always try to be one step ahead of the patient. Patients in the second stage need constant direction, and most of those in the final stage need to have practically everything done for them. It is important to be well organized and to have all necessary items handy before one begins any part of the daily routine, such as eating or bathing. For example, it is dangerous to leave Hughes in the kitchen alone, since he might turn on the gas, pick up a sharp knife, or swallow something inedible. My procedure, therefore, is to have his food ready on his plate before bringing him into the kitchen. Every little detail can be important in the care of an AD patient.

The caregiver has to be prepared to shift gears and move from one task to another. Being well organized can help to eliminate stress. Also, being able to proceed with a certain amount of confidence and assurance is essential to establishing a daily regimen with and for the patient. The unspoken feelings we emit will actually speak much louder than anything we say, and AD patients know when we are adrift in indecision as to what to do next. Throughout the years that Hughes has had AD, the two most stressful and difficult times of day have been in the morning when I wake him and get him up, and at night when I give him his supper and get him ready for bed. The morning and evening procedures have changed and evolved as he has progressed in the disease. In many ways his care in this present stage, though more physical, is less stressful than in earlier stages. This is partly because I have a routine but also because I have become more accepting, more experienced, and more confident. As Steven Zarit points out, "The severity of the disease does not necessarily correlate with the degree of burden experienced."[2]

At the time of diagnosis, if the family does not decide to institutionalize the patient, it is imperative that diagnosing physicians recommend a name, a phone number, a brochure or other printed information for family members who want to inquire about training in the management of the patient at home. Families need time to internalize the diagnosis, to learn about AD, and to explore all the options open to them. It is unconscionable today that doctors would diagnose AD without giving the family at the very least some small bit of information about where to go for help.

Unfortunately, most of the literature on AD is about the difficulties families face after the diagnosis of a loved one. The story of one family's successful home management of a patient might provide some hope and encouragement to a beginning caregiver. The several chapters of the Alzheimer's Association could develop brochures that introduce AD families and tell briefly how they manage the home care of the patient. For example, a single, middle-aged daughter could explain how she continues to take care of her mother by enrolling her in an adult day-care center while the daughter works at a full-time job. Or a retired spouse could relate her or his story of managing the AD patient at home. These could be stories of patients in various stages of the disease. Such brochures could be distributed by the chapters to local doctors' offices, complete with the phone number of an Alzheimer's Association help line. Beginning caregivers could be spared untold stress and heartache if given even this minimum of information, reinforcement, training, and counseling immediately after the diagnosis.[3]

When the patient reaches the stage of needing twenty-four-hour care, someone has to take charge and put daily procedures in place. As a caregiver, I find there is always a more efficient, productive and less stressful way of taking care of Hughes. Corporations know there is always a better way of accomplishing a given task, and they pay efficiency experts thousands of dollars to find new ways of using less time and energy in making a better product. I find myself pushed into becoming my own efficiency expert, especially in those periods when I am ill or very tired. The results are evident in the difference between how little time I have to put into Hughes's care today as compared to those early laborious and tedious days when he first needed twenty-four-hour care. In the morning it takes less than an hour and a half to get Hughes up and ready for the day. At night it once took two to four hours just to get him ready for bed; today it takes less than thirty minutes.

I am continually looking for more efficient ways of attending to his needs. I can now say that Hughes is often the least of my difficulties, primarily because my resistance to caring for him is so much lessened. Often it is not so much the tasks themselves as our resistance to them that causes us stress and wears us down.[4] Of course, Hughes himself is now less resistant, more passive, and more sedentary. I still experience some stress, but his care has become a built-in part of my daily routine. It is unexpected outside pressures—a phone call, a writing deadline, a speaking engagement, an unplanned trip, or a family crisis—that cause the greatest stress.

PROCEDURES IN THE BEGINNING STAGE

The beginning stage is a time when the caregiver develops inner procedures rather than outer ones. At this point the patient may or may not have been diagnosed and is still able to take care of her- or himself, but the caregiver and people closest to the patient have begun to detect short-term memory loss and personality changes. This is when the caregiver who wants to give home care a trial begins to develop and cultivate a new level of patience and understanding.

It was very difficult to stand by helplessly and watch Hughes take four hours to get ready for bed. It took him much longer to do everything in the beginning stage, but he could finally complete the task. He could bathe, shave, and dress himself; cook a meal and feed himself; mow, rake, and water the grass; dig dandelions; drive the car. He could do everything he had done before—but much more slowly. Even before I knew he had AD,

I had to be patient and spend a great deal of time waiting for him to finish the simplest task. The last household job Hughes undertook and completed was in 1987, when he replaced two pieces of tile in the bathroom. It took him three months, but the pieces fit perfectly when he finished.

In the beginning stage, then, I was something like a valet or butler, anticipating and supplying his needs. If we had an appointment, I made sure everything he needed to get ready for it was at his fingertips. Before AD, Hughes had waited on me. Now it was I who got ready first, brought the car around to the front, and stood by while he finished dressing.

PROCEDURES IN THE SECOND STAGE

After AD was diagnosed in early 1988, I realized that I had to begin instituting a regimen for Hughes's care. It made sense to start the procedures with the beginning of the day. He was often most alert in the morning after a night's rest, but even though he could still do many things for himself, he was slowly but steadily approaching the need for constant care. Yet because he still had brief intervals of lucidity, I often felt emotionally like a yo-yo. One moment he was off into the land of AD, and the next he had that light of recognition in his eyes, and I was once again his wife and we were a couple. But those brief interludes became too costly. They pulled me back into a world that was in fact gone. I realized that for my own healthy survival I had to develop a matter-of-fact attitude toward his rational periods. I could not afford to be lured back; I had to stay with my center and move forward with a plan for our survival. Giving up those last lingering bits of his lucidity was perhaps the most painful thing I had to do.

SOUNDS AND SIGHTS

I did, however, try several methods of assisting his memory. Our son Eric had often chided me for my resistance to learning the use of even the simplest of electronic equipment. He told me many times, "Ma, come into the twentieth century!" One day I thought there must be a way to put some of this electronic gadgetry to work helping us with AD patients. First, I interviewed Hughes on videotape, asking him about his life and beliefs. Next, I compiled a memorabilia book of family pictures, Hughes's writings, and newspaper clippings about him. In addition, our daughter Nena and her husband, Michael, made an hour-long videotape of their life in San Francisco, always addressing Hughes directly. Our daughter-in-law Chris, Cedric's wife, also made a videotape of their family in Oregon. In 1988 I took and passed the training course in using video equipment owned by public access cablevision and then made an hour-long documentary about Hughes and AD, which aired for the first time in 1989.

It also came to me to record the story of Hughes's life and let him listen to it. In 1988 I decided to begin his day by playing the audio tape of his life just as he was awakening. It began "Your name is Hughes Hannibal Shanks" and went on to give our address and phone number. Here is an abbreviated version of the twenty-minute tape:

"You have lived in this house since 1965, when you moved your family from Kansas City, Kansas, to Lincoln, Nebraska. For protection against possible attack, you slept in the bathtub on a board for a week before you moved your family into this house because you wanted to be sure the White neighbors would not harm your family.

"You have painted every wall and ceiling of this house many times. You and I textured the upstairs bedrooms. You laid the carpet downstairs and upstairs. You put the linoleum down in the kitchen. You carpeted the stairs. . . . You built a wall-to-wall bookcase in the dining room. You tiled the upstairs bathroom. You put a ceiling in the basement, and you put walls up in the basement. You have worked very hard to make your home comfortable and pleasant and attractive for me and for our children. All our children are grown now, however, and gone and living on their own. This is the only house we have lived in since we moved to Lincoln, Nebraska.

"You, Hughes Hannibal Shanks, were born in Palestine, Arkansas, on September 17, 1919. Your mother and father are now dead. Your father, Charles Shanks, died in 1957. Your mother, Susie Shanks, died in 1988. Your brother Asa is in his seventies and lives in St. Louis. He does not live in Lincoln. He is not here in your home with you. You also often think that your oldest sister, Emily, is here in our home, but Emily is well into her seventies, and she does not live here with us. She lives in Chicago with her husband. You live in Lincoln, Nebraska, . . . with me, your wife, Lela Nuna Knox Shanks. We have been married since Thanksgiving Day in 1947. I am from Oklahoma, and my mother and father are now dead. My brother, Johnnie, is also dead. My sister, Claudine, and her daughter, Claudette, and Johnnie's son, Leland, are my only living relatives.

"You, Hughes Shanks, have five children. Ronald is your oldest child. He lives in New Jersey . . . with his daughter, Stacey. Nena is our oldest child and our oldest daughter. She lives in San Francisco with her husband, Michael Lewis. She was born on your birthday and we called her your birthday present. Cedric, our oldest son, lives in La Grande, Oregon, with his wife, Chris, and their two children: Carrie . . . and Christopher. Cedric was born on May 22; he was our spring flower. Shela lives in New York City with her husband, Jim, and their two children, Orpheus and Zenith. . . . We drove to New York City when Orpheus was born, and then when Orpheus was three and one-half he came to Lincoln, Nebraska, and stayed a month with us. And when Zenith was born . . . you and I took the train to New York City, and we stayed with Shela and Jim and Orpheus and Zenith for about a week. Shela we always called our valentine, since she was born February 15. And then there is Eric who is our youngest. He lives in Lincoln, Nebraska. He is our only child still living in Lincoln, Nebraska, but he does not live here at home. Eric was born July 7. We called him our firecracker.

"In April 1988 you were diagnosed as having Alzheimer's disease. Because of your memory loss, most of the time you do not know me, Lela, your wife. You often think I am one of your sisters or one of your brothers or somebody that you grew up with. And you often ask me strange questions like, 'Did I know you in St. Louis?' or 'Did I know you at Union Memorial [Church]?' It is very difficult for me when you don't know me. . . .Every day now you ask me to take you to the 'other Lincoln,' but dear one, there is no other Lincoln. Because of your memory loss you have forgotten what our home looks like. But this is our home. This is the only home that we have that I can take you to. So you and I have to trust in life for what we cannot understand.

"I am Lela, your wife. I am here to take care of you as long as I am physically and mentally able to do so. I pray to be able to do so. But you have to cooperate with me. . . . I believe we can make it so long as we trust in life. Has life not always taken care of you? And life will take care of us now. . . . When you were a little child growing up in St. Louis selling newspapers on the streets, a little eight- or nine- or ten-year-old kid selling newspapers, didn't life take care of you? When you hoboed to Chicago, an eighteen- or nineteen-year-old kid, out on your own, no money, no place to stay, didn't life take care of you? When you needed an overcoat, wasn't an overcoat provided for you? When your ship got bombed and you had shrapnel coming out of your legs, didn't life take care of you? Every time you moved from another town, didn't life take care of you? Remember you have survived a war; you survived the Depression. . . . You and I have a legacy of life taking care of us. . . . And I know life has not forsaken us now."

After repeating his full name and address, the tape concluded, "You have lived here since 1965. This is the only home you have. There is no other

Lincoln to take you to. There is no other home to take you to. Your mother and father are now dead. This is your home. I am your wife, Lela, and I am here doing everything I can to take care of you, Hughes Shanks. I am your wife, Lela. I love you." Sometimes I watched Hughes listening to the tape. He would often smile and talk back to it.

Also, when he awoke every morning, the wall he faced was filled with memorabilia from his life. Our son-in-law Michael and our daughter Nena made three large posters labeled in big letters. "Family Tree of Hughes Shanks" had pictures of his mother and father and a picture of Hughes with his siblings, taken (before AD) at his mother's ninetieth birthday celebration. "Children of Hughes Shanks" had a panel for each of our five children and their families. "Attention Hughes H. Shanks" had a picture of Hughes in bed, and it read: "You are in your bedroom right now at [your home] in Lincoln, Nebraska. This is the only earthly home you have to go to. Your mother and father are dead. Signed: Lela (your wife)." In addition to the tape and posters, I started Hughes's morning by placing in full view a sign with the day of the week written in big letters.

HUGHES'S BOOK OF PROCEDURES

In 1989, when Hughes was in the second stage and could no longer be left alone, I wrote a book of procedures—a kind of working manual or detailed guide for family members and sitters to follow whenever I had to be away. I included a table of contents and numbered the pages for quick and easy referral, since timeliness is often critical in AD patient care, especially for a new caregiver. I wrote the information by hand and put it in a looseleaf notebook. Our early sitters were all laypeople with no previous experience or knowledge about what to do for a person who is demented (to date, I have not used a professional nursing service for Hughes's care in our home). Doubtless, some were afraid of what he might do to them, as I was in the beginning. Thus, I organized the book both to specify Hughes's needs, and to answer the direct inquiries new sitters had made. That determined the order in which topics were presented. I often followed the language of the sitters' questions in phrasing the information, and I used repetition for emphasis, since the caregivers were novices. As Hughes progressed in the disease, I continued to update sections as necessary to fit his changing needs.

When our son Cedric came in 1990 to take care of his father for a week, I sent the book to him beforehand; this gave him some advance reassurance about being his dad's caregiver. Afterward, Cedric told me, "It would have been flat out hard for me to know what to do and how to proceed, especially when he was being difficult, without that book. I was also able to stay constant with his schedule by referring to it." Likewise, when Eric kept his dad two or three days a week during this difficult period, he always asked, "Where's that book?"

Some in-home caregivers refuse to leave a loved one during the most active and difficult stages of AD; they fear that no substitute caregiver will know what to do. But preparing simple instructions tailor-made for each patient can alleviate some of the primary caregiver's anxieties and fears as well as assist the substitute. Support groups of the Alzheimer's Association could encourage members by including in their agenda time for helping caregivers write their own personalized books of procedures. In order for such a project to be successful, however, it is important to stress to caregivers at the outset that one does not have to be a writer to put down on paper in one's own words the needs of a loved one.

Here are excerpts from the notebook I kept in 1989. The topics are presented in a somewhat more straightforward, less personal sequence to maximize the usefulness of the information to readers of this book—but I begin with the first question that family members always asked.

Will He Know Me? He may know you some of the time. Whether he knows you or not will not interfere with your ability to care for him, as he will be going on his instinct and feelings when he is with you. Most of the time he does not know me, but this does not prevent him from cooperating. He will respond to his environment.[5] If you are hostile, he will feel it. If you are kind, he will feel that. If you take charge, he will know this, also. This will give him the security he needs, as he always feels so insecure—like something is missing. (And it is!) Your feelings for him and your being in charge will see you through. The important thing is that *you* know who *he* is.

Appearance versus Behavior. It is very deceiving to look at Hughes and think of him as demented. His outer appearance is still the same. He looks very much like any "normal" person. Be aware: It is very easy for this to throw you. His manner is still the same. He thinks he is talking about important issues, that he knows exactly what he is talking about, and that he is in complete command of himself, you, and the situation.

He will suddenly ask you a question. Often the question is nonsensical. The best procedure is to redirect whatever you say to a subject he can respond to with some remaining memory. For example, ask him, "Did you ever learn to swim?" or any of those questions under *Ways to Distract Him* [below]. I usually ignore his nonsensical questions, but this is something that comes with time and experience. Even I can still be caught off guard because his manner is the same as always. He looks you right in the eye, and he is so confident that he knows what he is talking about.

Remember: No matter how intelligent he might look or sound, you are in charge of a person who is now demented. Ignoring this fact can cause untold stress to you and to Hughes.[6]

One minute he may be cordial and the next minute hostile. (This may be because one minute he knows you and the next minute he thinks you are an impostor.) When he gets hostile, I ignore him or leave the room or change the subject. If you leave the room and he does not see you for a few minutes, he may remember you when you return, or his mood may have changed in your absence.

His personality is pleasant and cooperative 75 percent of the time. He is considerate within his understanding, but when he is confused, he does not cooperate. This takes place most often in the evening and at night. He is generally cooperative in the morning.

Hiding Items. He will hide anything.

When he takes his shoes off, it is wise to discreetly put them in the back room out of sight. Give him his house shoes instead. Otherwise, he might hide them. The back room is "off limits" to him, as that is where medications, notions, cleaning agents, and his underwear and socks are kept.

His favorite hiding places are under his pillows and mattress. He also hides objects behind chairs, couches, drapes, dressers; on high shelves and windowsills; and in the bookcase.

I usually try to get his coat and hat and put them in a back room out of sight so that he cannot hide them. (He will not try to leave the house without his hat and coat.)

If he asks about his shoes or coat and hat, I say, "Oh, they are in a safe place."

Accusations. He will accuse you of anything! You may be eating and he will suddenly say, "Why did you take my meat?" It is best either to ignore him or to say pleasantly, "Have you finished your dinner?" or "Is your dinner okay?" or "Finish your dinner."

He talks all the time, but most of what he says is not connected. Still, it is important to listen and to pay attention to him, remembering he is now demented.

Saying "No." He will say "no" to everything, but he will still respond positively. Try to proceed as if he did not say "no," unless physical contact is involved. When you are trying to get him to do something, he often responds best to a challenge, such as "Do you know how to take off your shirt?" (Always remove dirty clothes from the bathroom, as he often puts them right back on if they are in sight.)

Body Language. Because of aphasia, he cannot always express what his needs are, so you sometimes have to rely on body language. He may

> touch his stomach or groin area when he needs to sit on the toilet;
> touch his chest when he has indigestion (I give him two antacids for an upset stomach);
> touch his head when he wants to brush his hair.

Dizziness. The doctor said brain deterioration causes his dizziness. To date, his dizziness has always come when he first wakes up. It seems to occur every two to three months for a few days. When you go in his bedroom to get him up, ask him how he feels. He has always told me when he felt dizzy. Also, I could see it as he would hardly be able to stand up alone. If he says he is dizzy when he awakens, please give him one tablet of meclizine while he is sitting on the bed. He takes it three times a day. The dizziness usually stops in two or three days.

Then help him to the bathroom to urinate. Afterward, help him to wash his face and to brush his teeth. Then help him back to bed. On these days I let him stay in bed fifteen to thirty minutes longer. When he is less dizzy, I get him up and start his daily procedures.

If he was dizzy on Monday, then on Tuesday be alert to helping him to the bathroom when he awakens, just in case. After about the third day the dizziness subsides.

Medications. When he will not take his medication, please do not push it. Drop it for a few minutes and try later. On a second try he often takes it. Never leave his medication with him, as you cannot tell what he will do with it.

His medication consists of the following:

> one baby aspirin in the morning with breakfast (to prevent strokes);
> two tablets, three times a day, of ergoloid mesylates (to stimulate his brain), which do not have to be taken with meals;
> one tablet of meclizine three times a day as needed for dizziness, and this does not have to be taken with meals, but the meclizine may make him drowsy.

His medications are in the blue pill box in the left kitchen cabinet over the sink.

The Importance of Taking Charge. You have to look beyond his physical appearance and accept that you are with a man who has the abilities of a three- or four-year-old child. He needs direction for practically everything he does. It is very common, however, for AD patients to call upon all their remaining abilities to "show off" and to "put on for company."[7] You will be like company to him, so he may be able to perform some tasks that I say he is no longer able to do. There may also be times when you need to say:

"You have a responsibility to cooperate with me."
"I am here for you, and I expect you to do your part."
"I am doing my job. You also have a job. Your job is to cooperate."

The Value of Repetition. Like most human beings, Hughes can still learn from repetition. Sometimes I repeat the same instructional statement over and over again. Many times he may be looking straight at you as you speak, but his brain will be hearing other words. So it may take two or three times for him to finally "hear" what you are saying.

Ways to Distract Him. Distractions provide a positive alternative to engaging in a power struggle with the patient. Distractions are especially important when physical confrontations might be involved.

Call to him and say, "Hughes! Eric is on the phone." Sometimes I call Eric or my friend Cynthia and ask them to talk with him.

Sometimes I dial our own phone number and let it ring. He always answers it and "talks" for long periods of time.

Ask him a question from his earliest past, such as "Hughes, can you swim?" "Did you ever go to church?" "Did you have a brother named Asa?" "Did you ever sell newspapers?" "Were you ever a Boy Scout?"

Play a videotape of him or a family member. He always seems fascinated watching himself on television. Sometimes he thinks it is his older brother, Asa.

Get his memorabilia book and ask him, "Have you seen this?" He will spend hours looking at it.

Give him a basket of clothes to fold. (If necessary, empty a drawer of clean clothes into the basket for folding.)

Take him to the table and give him a deck of playing cards and ask him to put them in numerical order.

Sometimes he will respond to questions about his religious beliefs. He will usually join with you if you begin saying the Lord's Prayer or the Twenty-third Psalm.

He will also join you in singing.

What Helps Him Most. Constant reassurance

that he is safe,
that "everything" is in place,
that "the children" are okay,
that the doors are locked,
that you love him.

He may ask about his mom and dad, his children, his siblings, or me. Tell him, "Oh, they are fine." Mainly he needs to know everything is okay, since everything in his mind is disconnected.

Be firm when you are trying to get him to do something. But if he still refuses, leave it for a few minutes and then start over.

Singing quietly sometimes helps to calm him down.

Morning Procedures. Play the audio tape of the story of his life.

Give him one-half glass of juice in a plastic tumbler and tell him it is time to get up. He will need a little time, as he will be befuddled. Then tell him it is time to get up and brush his teeth and wash up or bathe as the case may be. Constantly reassure him that his clothes are "right here," but keep them out of the bathroom, as he may hide them or try to put them on before washing up.

If you are giving him a morning bath, run his water. You will have to tell him how to take his night clothes off or assist him. (Be sure to shut the door to his bedroom, since he will sometimes try to go back to bed. When he does this and will not get up after a reasonable time, I begin very slowly removing his bed covers, piece by piece. I put them in the dining room out of sight. Once his covers are gone, he gets up.)

When he finishes washing up, he may need guidance in putting on each article of clothing.

Be sure that you put his glasses on for him. If you hand them to him, he will not know what to do with them.

Prepare his toothbrush with toothpaste and show him how to brush his teeth. Afterward, take a chair into the bathroom, have him sit down, and put his shoes and socks in front of him. He can usually put them on.

Next tell him, "Now we shave." Help him to stand and spray the shaving cream in his right palm. Take two fingers of his left hand and put them in the cream and tell him to put it on his face. He usually catches on and does it. Put his razor in his left hand and motion to him what to do. Again something triggers and he begins. When he finishes, I help him cup his hands and pour aftershave in them, making sure he does not drink it.

While he is shaving, I fix breakfast. I place his plate on the kitchen counter in the same place each time he eats. When he finishes, I help him brush his teeth again and assist him with hand lotion.

On day-care days I get his hat and coat if it is cold and tell him it is time to go. (It is important for the caregiver to be ready to leave when Hughes has finished eating in order to keep the momentum going, so that he does not have a chance to sit down and settle in.) Tell him, "They are waiting for you at the church." That is what he calls the day care. If he refuses to cooperate when you ask him to go with you to the car, try one or more of the following:

See if his shoes are untied.

Take him by the hand to the bathroom; he may need to use it.

Give him some tissues; he may want to blow his nose.

Tell him that what he is looking for is already in the car or that you have it.

Ask him to go out and get the mail; always have your key ready to act quickly.

Caution in the Car. Hughes's depth perception is distorted because of his brain deterioration, so he is often afraid of having an accident when he is riding in the car. Be prepared for him to suddenly exclaim anything to you. He often says, "Turn here! Turn here!" "No, no! Go in that lane!" "Take a left, take a left!" "Where do you think you are going?" "Man, I want to go home!" "Stop the car! I'll walk home!"

It is best not to reply to these remarks. I try to drive carefully and to reassure him by saying, "Everything is all right. You are safe. You are okay." When I can, I also pat him reassuringly on the leg. A few times I shouted, "Shut up!" and he did!

Activities after Day Care. Tell him, "Hang your hat and coat up." (At a later time, I put his wraps out of his sight.) I tell him, "Brush your teeth and wash your face," assisting him. He might need to spend time sitting on the toilet. If dinner is not ready or if you have taken him out to eat, put the playing cards on the dining room table and ask him to put them in order;

or give him the United States puzzle; or bring one of his books and ask him to read you a story. If you do not direct him when he is home, he may get into anything, because he wants to help but seldom understands how anymore. Most nights he will occupy himself with what you give him until time for bed.

Areas That Are Off Limits. For his safety, the parts of the house where I keep the liquids he might drink and the objects he would surely hide are off limits. They include

> the kitchen (except for eating),
> my room (the back room),
> the basement (usually he acts afraid to go down there),
> upstairs.

He has his bedroom and the dining and living rooms for his space. Anytime he is quiet in another room, you need to check on him.

Coffee and Other Beverages. He should not have liquids after his dinner.

He may say he wants a cup of coffee or he may offer to make you some, but he is just being courteous. He drinks coffee only in the morning at day care. He never drinks coffee at home anymore because it keeps him awake. Whenever he talks about coffee, I change the subject.

Bedtime Procedures. The best time to start getting him ready for bed is between seven-thirty and eight-thirty. The later you wait, the harder it is to get him to cooperate. If you wait until nine o'clock, he is often much more disoriented, and giving him a bath is much more difficult.

If the television is on, it is best to distract him and then turn it off and say, "Time for bed." If this does not work, discreetly take all three light bulbs out of the lamps in the sitting room and disconnect their electric cords. Turn the light on in his bedroom. With the living area darkened, direct him to his bedroom. He will try to turn the lamp switches back on, but when he is unsuccessful, he will come to the light in his bedroom. A flashlight comes in handy after I remove the light bulbs.

Get his clean underwear and pajamas out and tell him he must now take his clothes off to take a bath. (But do not leave his clean clothes in the bathroom before he is in the tub, or he will hide them.) Ask him, "Can you take your shirt off?" "Do you know how to take off your pants?"

Run his bath water, put his washcloth in the tub, and show him his soap. He still understands how to get into the tub, and he can bathe himself.

Give him as much privacy as possible. At the same time it is necessary to stay close by, praising him and encouraging him to wash all body parts. If you have not gotten his dirty clothes, quickly remove them when he washes his head.

When he finishes his bath, tell him to step out and hand him his towel. He likes to stand in the tub and dry off as he did before AD, but that is too dangerous, so assist him out as you hand him his towel. When he is out of the tub, put his deodorant on. If you let him do it, he sometimes puts it on his hair and face. He can usually dress himself, but he may need assistance. He likes to clean the tub. You put the cleanser in and give him a cloth.

After he gets in bed, I read with him from one of his devotional books and then we say the Lord's Prayer.

I take his eyeglasses off while distracting him by asking, "Did you ever swim?" Otherwise, he will sleep in his glasses or hide them. Once in bed, he sleeps soundly except for getting up maybe once during the night to use the bathroom.

Additional Tips. When you are trying to get him to take his clothes off and get in the tub, ask him, "Are you in the tub?" rather than "Do you have your clothes off?" Asking him about the "next step" seems to stimulate him into action.

Sometimes he will not leave the bathtub faucets alone. He will turn them on and off over and over again. I believe he wants to start a bath, but he does not know how to proceed beyond turning the faucets on, and he refuses my help. If it is not time for a bath, I go to the basement and turn off all water to the house, unknown to him. [Note: This was before I had shut-off valves installed in the bathroom.] When he can no longer get the water to run, he loses interest.

When you put his glasses on or give him his pants or shoes, he may say they are not his. I just say matter-of-factly, "Put your pants on," and I never speak to what he is saying.

One cannot reason with dementia. But love can understand.

If you take him out among people, be prepared for him to act familiar with everyone. I always make sure to lead him away when he starts talking to children, since his friendliness might be misunderstood. He will flirt with women and say to anyone, "Don't I know you from St. Louis?" It is wise to put his pin reading "Alzheimer's Patient" on his lapel. This will explain his behavior.

New caregivers feel so helpless in the face of AD, especially in the second stage. I cannot say for sure how much the structure I worked out helped

Hughes, but these procedures and routines helped me through the most difficult periods of his care.

PROCEDURES IN THE THIRD STAGE

Although Hughes's mentality has deteriorated to that of an infant, he is much calmer now that he is probably entering the third stage. He still has fears, but he seems to feel much safer. He sleeps more during the day; the turbulent confusion, disorientation, and agitation of the second stage have all but disappeared. He is still confused and disoriented, but he seems to be more settled into it. He seems to go with the confusion now. And even though almost everything has to be done for him, he still has some important assets, chief among them his mobility; he continues to be a strong walker. Other assets include his general cooperativeness, his desire to be clean and neat, his personal warmth and charm, his cheerfulness, his great appetite, and his ability to feed himself most of the time. My goal is to reinforce his assets through the daily procedures.

On the days he goes to day care, I get him up about six-thirty in the morning and have him sit on the toilet. I hand him a cup of warm water or a cup of warm orange juice. He usually welcomes the cup I give him, as I say, "Here is your hot coffee." I check on him for the next fifteen or twenty minutes while he wakes up and eliminates. Each time I leave the bathroom, I always tell him, "I'll be right back, now don't leave me." This is my way of reassuring him and at the same time trying to tell him he is needed. By seven o'clock I can wash his face and begin shaving him, all while he is sitting on the toilet. I give him a magazine to hold so he won't interfere. Afterward, I stand him up for his washup. I encourage him to wash his hands while I am working with him. Once again this occupies his hands. When the washup is finished, I brush his teeth. Then I set him once again on the toilet and dress him there. I stand him up to pull up his undergarments and pants. I wash and lotion his hands and take him out into the dining room and put him in a straight chair. I give him a bowl of bite-sized pieces of fruit to eat until Eric comes to pick him up between eight and eight-thirty.

In the evening I pick Hughes up from the day-care center around five o'clock. When the weather is warm, I often park about a mile from the center and walk the rest of the way so that he can get the exercise of walking to the car. We have two busy intersections to cross, and the traffic sometimes frightens him. But I hang on to him tightly, constantly reassuring him that he is all right. In the winter when it is too cold and icy to walk outside, I take him two or three times each week to the state capitol building, where we walk twenty to thirty minutes. Three and a half times around the long corridors is about a mile. When we begin a walk, Hughes is unsure of what is happening. But I start by holding his hand or arm, steering him, and after a few strides something clicks in and he takes off. Throughout our marriage we loved taking long walks together. He always walked back and forth to work. He even walked in several Lincoln Senior Olympics before AD.

When we reach our car, it usually takes a while to get Hughes into it. Each time, it is as if he is learning how all over again. When we reach home, I have to wait for him to understand how to get out of the car. Sometimes I take his legs firmly but gently and swing them out of the car. Then he will stand up. I guide him to the back door and into the bathroom if he has not voided lately (this information is provided by the day-care staff). I remove his coat and hat and set him on the toilet. After washing his hands I take him to the kitchen to eat a light supper (the day-care center provides a full meal at noon). It is a great stress reducer for me to eat my supper and wash the dishes before I go to pick up Hughes. Then my time is free to assist him. I give him his evening medications, take him to the bathroom to brush his teeth, and guide him to the couch, where he sits with his papers and dolls until bedtime. Sometimes I throw the ball back and forth to him to wake him up.

At seven or seven-thirty I set Hughes on the toilet, remove his clothes, and put his undergarments and pajamas on. I take him to his bed and say our prayers. I kiss him good-night, and he always returns the kiss.

On Saturdays I take Hughes to day care at eleven-thirty, and he is at home on Sundays. On weekend mornings after I have gotten him up to void and washed his face and hands, I put him back in bed, propped on his backrest, and give him a bowl of fruit in bite-sized pieces. He feeds himself between naps. I tell him we are having a party.

SEVEN
Dealing with Problem Behavior

Understanding why AD patients act as they do can be a first step in dealing with problem behavior.[1] But even more important is understanding that we can choose our attitude for handling difficult behavior. As Holocaust survivor Viktor E. Frankl has stated; "If . . . one cannot change a situation that causes his suffering, he can still choose his attitude."[2] And the attitude we choose ultimately determines how we approach problems and how we solve them.[3] It sets the tone and influences the quality of our interactions with the patient. Attitude also determines the quality of our patient care.

Samuel Lipkin, a retired psychiatrist, brought his wife, who had AD, to the same day-care center Hughes attends. Dr. Lipkin took care of Pauline in their home for several years before her death. He told me, "Once I was able to get at my anger and my rage at having to be put into this position, . . . it just made my ability to cope with whatever problems Pauline was presenting, [to see each one] as a problem that needed to be solved and resolved. I approach each day with, 'Well, there is going to be a set of problems today concerning her, and whatever they are I'll find a solution for them.' And I take one day at a time in that fashion." Further, Dr. Lipkin explained, he realized that the quality of care he provided for his wife would depend not upon her or what she did but upon how he handled his emotions.[4] The patient cannot change back to his or her former self, but we so-called normal human beings can adapt and grow and develop new understandings.

Working with an AD patient demands a radically new response from us. We have to learn a new way and do a new thing. When we are in denial, we continue to try to relate to the patient in the old way, the usual and comfortable way; we also try over and over again to use reason and logic with the patient—all to no avail. Sometimes it takes years before we finally stop trying to talk the patient out of having the disease. Of course, we never want to completely give up our loved one as we knew her or him in the past, and we always want AD to go away. Our initial resistance to the disease is predictable and understandable; it is human and natural for us to be filled with the anger and rage referred to by Dr. Lipkin.[5]

But everything seems harder than it really is when we are resisting the present reality. Our determination to "talk" AD away, and to make the patient behave as before, closes the door to solutions. In our great despair, grief, and self-pity, we are often blinded to the possibility of creating a new life and a new world for ourselves and our loved one in spite of AD. Ralph Waldo Emerson said, "We cannot let our angels go. We do not see that they only go out that archangels may come in."[6] It is out of an accepting attitude that creative techniques are born.

Careproviding presents us with the challenge of a lifetime, and the hardest task many of us will ever face. But the extraordinary circumstances in which it places us are also opportunities to open up new frontiers in human development and understanding. It has been said that all the progress of humankind has been born out of hardship and pain, the tough circumstances of life. In our civilization there seems to be no limit to our pursuit of technology to develop the body. Records of physical endurance are made to be broken. Our son Eric is an endurance athlete. He has told me many times, "The benefits to the body from the self-improvement through exercise begin to diminish until there is no gain if an athlete reaches a level of competency and remains there." After more than a decade of experience with Hughes, I now believe this is also true of our inner and mental development. Certainly, our knowledge of inner and mental endurance in interpersonal relations has lagged light years behind that of our physical endurance. Albert Einstein said that with the splitting of the atom everything had changed except our thinking.[7] But as caregivers, lay or professional, we have to think the unthinkable and do the undoable in order to discover the creative techniques necessary for continually successful AD care.

In some ways, lay caregivers, despite their initial ignorance of AD, may have an advantage over the professionals. They have not been exposed to textbooks and lectures on what AD patients can and cannot do. Neither are they tied to certain models of care; rather, they fashion a model to fit the individual patient. For innovative and creative home caregivers, the field is wide open and the sky is the limit.

Fortunately, I had the example of a creative and confident mother; even in my greatest rage and anguish it never occurred to me that I would *not* be able to deal with Hughes's behavior or to find solutions to the problems we faced. Like Dr. Lipkin, I always knew that my patient's care would depend not upon what he said or did or did not do but upon how I handled my negative emotions and how creatively I dealt with his problem behavior.

VIOLENCE AND FORCE

When I talk to groups about AD, the most frequent question I get is about violence. Well-meaning people constantly ask about Hughes, "Is he violent?" in much the same tone as one might inquire of a dog owner, "Will he bite?" When I am asked if I think he might hurt me, I answer that he is probably in greater danger from me than I am from him.

I sometimes say Hughes reminds me of a gentle elephant in the way he stands quietly by while I manage him and handle his body. Sometimes I hold his hands as I try to get him to drink liquids. Once he asked falteringly, "May I have my hand back?" Since he is still strong and could doubtless knock me out with one blow, his asking for his hand recalls an elephant that accepts being tied by a rope.

To avoid accidental violence, I have found it wise to face Hughes when I want to touch any part of his body. I do not grab him from the back or side, because since he lives in a world of confusion, not knowing where he is or who I am, he might think he is being attacked and strike out to defend himself. I also try to avoid sudden movements toward him. I use my tone of voice and eye contact to communicate to him that he is safe with me.

To date, Hughes has rarely shown any violence toward me or anyone else to my knowledge. There were incidents of aggression when he was at the height of his second-stage confusion and disorientation, and I exhausted myself shouting out answers and directions he could no longer comprehend. Gradually and painfully I was able to stop reacting to his hostile and aggressive manner. I refused to feed into his negative mood and energy. My response to everything he said became a cheerful statement or question on an entirely different subject. In such an atmosphere his hostility and aggression quickly dissipated.

In the earlier stages of the disease, before I gained self-confidence in managing Hughes, I did not take chances. Whenever I was in doubt about his behavior, I left the room. I would go to my safe place in the upstairs bathroom and lock the door. Sometimes, when he looked or acted menacing, I would make sure there was some distance between us and then tell him forcefully, "Don't you dare touch me! Don't you ever try to hurt me!" I think my tone and volume startled and delayed him. Some caregivers have recounted incidents of a patient unexpectedly attacking and hitting the caregiver from behind, but this has never happened with Hughes—perhaps because I learned in the beginning stage to watch my back.

I heard a Benedictine sister who was also a nurse and had worked with

AD patients for several years say that when the patient becomes violent, there is usually a secondary cause: an infection (such as an inflamed bladder), or constipation, or pain somewhere.[8] I reiterate, it is my experience that the Alzheimer's patient responds instinctively to his or her emotional environment. If I am hostile, mean, and aggressive with Hughes, he reacts to protect himself. But when I am patient and accepting, kindness speaks a universal language and elicits kindness in return.

Because it is human and natural for any of us to resist force and to retaliate in the face of it, I believe it is possible for Hughes to become violent and to defend himself if I should strike out in anger at him and try to physically force him to do something he doesn't understand or want to do. (In his present stage of AD, of course, he is much slower to react to any action taken against him.) Alzheimer's patients are at the mercy of their caregivers, whether at home or in an institution. All decisions are made by someone else: when to get up; what and when to eat; whether face and hands are washed; when and how long to use the bathroom. The list is endless.

Unfortunately, the use of force as a means to an end is built into our American culture; we are a hurry-up, do-it-now, impatient society. As a nation, when things do not go our way, we often view force as an acceptable alternative. Force is what we know; consequently, although it is almost always nonproductive as a long-term solution, the use of force is common in nursing homes. According to OSCAR Report 18, 6 January 1994, 18 percent of all skilled nursing facilities and 16 percent of all nursing facilities in the United States at that time were in violation of the regulation prohibiting the use of physical restraints. And according to the National Citizens' Coalition for Nursing Home Reform, "Use of physical restraints in place of alternative methods of care is a major cause of incontinence, pressure ulcers, infections, fractures, dehydration and malnutrition."[9]

The times I have used force with Hughes have seldom had anything to do with him but have been, rather, the result of my own impatience, resentment, and anger. If I pull him out the door rather than wait for him to understand and come out on his own, for example, it is usually not because a few more minutes would create a time crisis but because I am impatient. Yet I always know immediately that I have regressed and taken a step backward. We cannot use force and be creative at the same time. Force cancels out creativity. It reinforces itself and makes everything harder every time we use it. Going beyond force and anger in human relationships is painful, but when we do, it is like cracking the "inner" sound barrier and entering a new dimension of consciousness. It is in this new dimension that the caregiver discovers the creative techniques that speak to the heart and needs of the AD patient.

INCONTINENCE

Even the most conscientious caregivers balk at dealing with incontinence in the AD patient. Many caregivers have told me they can tolerate the memory loss and subsequent bizarre behavior but not this. Like a little child, the AD patient may at times be likely to eliminate anywhere. In addition to his clothes closet, heat vent, washbasin, and bathtub, Hughes has used the corners of his bedroom, his bed, the floor next to his bed, and the bathroom floor. I have run the gamut of feelings from disbelief and anger to downright rage at having to clean up after such behavior. Yet I have not been able to come up with one satisfactory reason why I cannot keep him and his environment clean and live satisfactorily despite his incontinence. In fact, it seems incongruous that we have the capacity to develop technology for disposing of the bodily waste of our astronauts as they orbit the earth yet lack the capacity to cope with incontinence in our loved ones who live with us here on earth.

After I had to change Hughes and all his bedding three times in one night, I learned quickly to use draw-sheets and several pads on the mattress. Sometimes I also placed a large pad or diaper around Hughes's groin area in order to prevent soiling of the top sheet and blankets.

To solve the problem of Hughes urinating in his room, I have positioned his bed so that if he gets up, the only place he can go is into the bathroom, where the tile makes the floor easy to clean even if he makes a mistake. Cedric put up a partition that prevents him from climbing across his bed to the other side of the room.

I have found two schools of thought concerning the inevitability of incontinence in AD patients. The popular belief is that all or most AD patients will become incontinent as a normal part of the progression of the disease.[10] People who hold this belief generally recommend putting the patient in diapers when he or she begins to have accidents. Of course, once in diapers, the patient is treated as incontinent, and the expectation often becomes the reality.

A second group does not see it that way, however; these people believe that even as the disease progresses, the patient will remain continent if taken to the bathroom on a frequent and regular schedule. They do not view incontinence as inevitable for all or even most AD patients, and indeed, I know one patient in her nineties and others in their eighties who are still continent. Some AD day-care centers refuse to accept patients wearing diapers. In one such center, staff members routinely take patients to the restroom every two hours; according to the director, this enables the patients to remain continent.

Recently, I took Hughes to see his urologist. His first question to me was, "Why do you have him in diapers?" He told me Hughes would not need them if I took him to the bathroom every three to four hours. By this time, however, Hughes was trained to wear the diapers, although it had taken him two years to learn that he must now sit down every time he goes to the bathroom instead of standing to urinate. Still there are times when he tries to stand, almost always wetting on the diaper and on himself.

On the days Hughes is home, I do take him to the bathroom on a regular schedule, every three to four hours, and 75 percent of the time he does remain continent. According to the day-care staff, he is continent there most of the time so long as he is regularly taken to the bathroom. He generally remains continent most of the time at night as well if I get him up once or twice. When I do, he is usually cooperative and ready to void, but because I do not always feel like getting him up, I put two heavy diapers on him for the night.

REPETITIVE ACTS

Repetitious behavior is a direct result of short-term memory loss. In the beginning stage when Hughes asked the same question over and over again, I wanted to scream and sometimes did, but that was not a satisfactory solution. I learned that the best solution was for me to be quiet and not speak; instead, I wrote Hughes notes during that stressful period. He could still read them, and since he asked the same questions each day, I accumulated a set of stock answers that I flashed to his questions. By keeping silent I was better able to remain calm, to stay centered and meditate. I had learned from the sisters (chapter 8) that we are always more vulnerable when we are speaking than when we are silent. Hughes never questioned why I was communicating with him through signs.

When he hummed the same refrain ad infinitum, there were moments when I asked myself, "How can I stand this?" But I found solutions: ignoring him, removing myself from his environment, distracting him by leading him in singing, turning on music from the radio or television, asking him a question, or taking him for a walk.

Some patients also display repetitive body motions, as Blanche did (chapter 3). Some walk in place, marking time in one spot; others continually walk forward then backward, or in a circle.

SUNDOWNING

Even though Hughes was a great one for "sundowning"—pacing back and forth, getting more and more anxious and agitated as darkness fell— he was not destructive in the house, nor did he try to hurt me. His sundowning was not harming anything or anyone; the problem arose because I did not want him to do it. He was like a man in a trance, obsessed, unable to help himself, racing back and forth for several hours until he went to bed. He acted as if he did not even know I was there. Fortunately, both the repetitive acts and the sundowning happened before he began to wander off from home (see below), so my main solution was to remove myself from his environment. Each day I planned ahead what I would work on in the evening while he was sundowning, and when he started I gathered what I needed and went upstairs.

Problems at this stage often arise because caregivers try to restrain their patients physically. We caregivers in our great denial think that if we can just stop them from what they are doing, the disease will go away. Caregivers trained in the management of patients learn that, in time, this too will pass. As Hughes lost more and more of his memory, the sundowning disappeared, and a calm and a tranquillity came over him that continue today.

WANDERING

When patients' memories are gone, they lose the images of the world they knew and strike out in search of something, anything, recognizable. I know one caregiver whose husband was so determined to wander that she sometimes gave up trying to stop him and, instead, followed him in her car.

It is a mistake to underestimate what an AD patient might be able to do when seized by the urge to wander. At the day-care center, in addition to trying to get over the fence, some patients have tried to crawl under it. One man quietly and persistently unwound enough of the fence wire to make a hole almost large enough to go through.

My solutions to wandering have included putting an identification bracelet on Hughes; writing his name and address on his clothing; registering him with the police as an AD patient (the Alzheimer's Association sponsors, "Safe Return," a nationwide community-based program that enables local police departments to identify AD patients who are prone to wander); notifying homeowners and businesses along routes Hughes might walk that he is an AD patient and giving them my name and phone number; installing an alarm system on our outer doors; putting a gate and lock on his bedroom door.

ACCUSATIONS AND MOOD SWINGS

The best way to handle accusations is to ignore them. We cannot talk a patient out of having the symptoms of the disease—a hard lesson for caregivers to learn when we are in denial. I created enormous stress for myself by trying to argue with Hughes's wild accusations; he looked so normal when he accused me of "going to meet another man" every time I left the house without him. As I began to accept his dementia, however, I freed myself from trying to convince him he was wrong. Reasoning with an AD patient is like hitting one's head against a stone wall. To help myself get beyond denial, I repeated aloud over and over again, "My husband is demented. My husband is demented."

Patients will accuse caregivers and others of many things, especially of stealing their possessions and money. Before the patient reaches this stage, it is wise for the caregiver to arrange a durable power of attorney, since the patient is no longer competent to handle his or her financial and medical affairs. When Hughes was in this phase, I made sure the checkbooks were out of his reach.

In the first two stages of the disease, Hughes was prone to sudden outbursts of anger and frustration as well as accusation. His moods were very fickle, quickly changing back and forth between happy and sad or irate. One minute he knew me and was laughing, and the next minute he was angrily accusing me of being an impostor. I found it best to ignore him or to leave the room for a brief interval. I cannot even imagine the fear and anxiety Hughes must have felt when his memory was going and coming and changing like the wind. Now that most of his memory is gone, however, his anxieties appear to be almost nil.

HALLUCINATIONS

It is common for AD patients to hallucinate, seeing things, people, and animals that are not there. Here again, it is totally useless for caregivers to spend energy trying to talk them out of their hallucinations; they are real to the patient. At the same time, hallucinations should not be ignored if they are causing the patient great anxiety and stress. There were times I could not get Hughes out of the house until I "picked up the baby" and told him we would not leave the baby alone but take it with us.

Once I accepted Hughes's concerns and treated him with respect, it did not take much to allay his fears. It is important to validate patients' feelings and treat them like human beings. Barbara Sand, a registered nurse and member of the national board of the Alzheimer's Association, whose father had AD, recounts an incident she witnessed while working on an acute care ward. She tells of a bedridden man who continued to cry out that a fire was under his bed, a fire was under his bed, over and over again. Finally, a nurse took a glass of water and threw it under the bed, saying, "There. I put the fire out." The distressed old man said with great relief, "Oh, thank you."

DRIVING AND THE AD PATIENT

At his second diagnosis, I was advised to stop Hughes from driving, and I knew I had to. Yet confronting him about it did not seem wise, since he was still lucid a great deal of the time. But in the second stage of the disease, experiencing his greatest confusion, anxiety, and hostility, he started abruptly bringing the car to a halt in the middle of a block, wondering where he was going. As a driver, he had become a hazard to himself and to others.

It came to me to get his ring of keys surreptitiously, remove his car key, and replace it with a key that resembled it but would not fit into the ignition. I purchased a new key from our local locksmith after explaining what I needed. Thereafter, when Hughes tried to start the car and could not get the key to fit, I would say, "Well, I will just drive," and we would exchange places. Hughes knew he needed a different key and spoke of getting one, but he no longer remembered how to go to the locksmith. Eventually, he stopped getting into the car on the driver's side, and the problem of his driving was solved without a confrontation.

Once I am able to get beyond my own anger and my resistance to Hughes's behavior at that moment, I am able to see a solution. I continue to find that the mastery of self is the mastery of problems.

PART THREE
Surviving the Stress of Caregiving

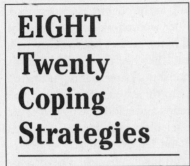

EIGHT
Twenty Coping Strategies

It is well documented that extended periods of AD caregiving in the home by a family member create high levels of emotional stress for the caregiver.[1] Studies also show that the determining factor of the outcome physically and mentally for the caregiver is his or her attitude and approach to life.[2] As noted in the preceding chapter, I soon recognized that the kind of care I gave Hughes would depend not upon him but upon me and how I handled my emotions. How does this make a difference? What are these emotional stresses and how do we cope with them?

The emotions most frequently associated with caregiving are negative emotions, since this is a job most of us do not want and did not choose; rather, we were chosen. In addition to anger, rage, and hate we experience resentment, bitterness, guilt, shame, embarrassment, fear, anxiety, depression, sorrow, self-pity, grief, impatience, blame. Beginning caregivers are flooded with a constant stream of uncertainties about the present and future. There are the endless "What if" questions: "How will I manage?" "Will there be enough money?" "Will I have to go bankrupt?" "Will we lose our home?" These concerns must be confronted on some level by every AD family.

For some caregivers, the first major struggle is to accept intellectually that these negative emotions in fact reside inside of us. In my own life I spent at least the first thirty years denying that I had any negative emotions. I especially denied having any hate. As a child growing up in the church, I learned early that bad people had hate and good people had love, and I wanted to be one of the good people. I do not remember ever being told that it was human and natural to have both good and bad feelings. Consequently, I grew up burying my anger and hate—pretending I was above them and that they were not there.

Fortunately, before I was forty I became aware of my negative feelings and also recognized my ability to destroy myself and others if I continued to deny their existence. I believe each of us has threads and themes in our lives that lead us to moments of greater self-consciousness and can prepare us to cope effectively with each new hardship. Hughes always said every difficult experience is preparing us to face a new level of difficulty. I did not willingly initiate this inward-looking process, however. It began as one of the most unusual experiences of my life.

In 1962, when Hughes and I were working in the civil rights movement, I met Sharon and Orpha, two reclusive older women whom I called "the sisters," since they were siblings. They lived in the greater Kansas City area. I was a guest on a local radio talk show, and they heard me tell about my experiences with racial prejudice and discrimination. Later that night Sharon called me at home and invited me to come to their house for lunch. Over the phone they spoke as if we were old friends and had known each other all our lives (I knew the familiar air of the telephone salesperson, and this was something different). I was intrigued and felt immediately drawn to them. At the same time, I was frightened and suspicious. I had never spoken with anyone who in the first phone conversation seemed to accept me so completely even though we had never met. My suspicions were further aroused when they confirmed that they were White women. I was thirty-five years old, and this was the first time I could remember a woman who was White inviting me to come inside her home for lunch.

It was also a time when we were receiving racist hate calls and anonymous death threats through the mail. Hughes and I speculated that maybe these women were plants for the FBI, which was at that time investigating us. Or even worse, maybe they were Communists! Being Communist was what the FBI was accusing us of, but I had never met a Communist. So I was polite in our first phone conversations but declined Sharon's invitation to their home. The sisters would not take no for an answer, however; day after day and week after week they continued to call and talk to both Hughes and me. After about four weeks of these ongoing phone conversations, we reluctantly agreed that it was safe for me to go for a visit.

When I first walked into Sharon and Orpha's home, I remember being overwhelmed by a feeling of magnificent beauty and peace. I felt as if I had come home, as if I belonged there. I said to myself, "This must be what heaven looks like." I thought it was the outer trappings, the furniture and decorations. Since I was not yet in touch with my feelings on a conscious level, the physical world was largely where I looked for explanations and interpretations of everything. The sisters later told me that their furniture had come from a Salvation Army store.

I have never met anyone before or since like them. Sharon, the leader of the two, had once been a model. Her ex-husband had worked in the Truman administration, and she had been a part of the Washington social scene. All her life, she said, she had known that there was a world of reality beyond the physical but had never found anyone who understood what she was talking about. She said she experienced deep inner pain and misery until she began the full-time practice of prayer and inner development. Orpha had always been a housewife. After her husband died, she and Sharon decided to live together permanently. They spent their days and nights deliberately and consciously studying and meditating to develop their inner life. They spoke of it as "working out their own maturity." I had read of nuns and monks who lived in monasteries and devoted their lives to prayer and contemplation, but Sharon and Orpha were not members of any religious order or denomination. They were laypeople like us. They never left their home, yet they were in touch with events and people all over the world.

It was through our discussions on race and prejudice that the sisters introduced me to the broad picture of the human condition, which spans all races. Before meeting Sharon and Orpha I had viewed my entire life through the prism of race. One had to, in order to survive growing up in a legally separated society. As a child, I could not afford to forget that I was a Negro. In fact, away from home, my physical safety depended upon knowing "my place," where I could and could not go, what I could and could not do. Every facet of my life was influenced if not totally controlled by my racial identity. Over a period of years after meeting the sisters, however, I reluctantly began to see that part of my humanity which extends beyond race, including my own human depravity and negativity.

Sharon and Orpha taught me that we live in two worlds: the outer world of the physical and the material; and the inner world of the mind, the soul, and the spirit. Their watchword was "Nothing availeth from without. All is from within." I learned that it is through our inner life that we are able to transcend, first, our individual, inner human depravity and, second, life's adversities—those outer circumstances and events, like AD, that are beyond our control.

The sisters worked with me for fourteen years. They wrote me hundreds of letters giving specific instructions on the development of an inner life. Both are now deceased, but it was through their guidance that I began this lifelong process of self-confrontation and inner development. And it is from the sisters' direct influence that I have developed coping strategies for reducing the emotional stresses I face every day in caring for Hughes. The essence of these twenty strategies was already a part of my life. I have given them specificity for caregivers. They include both inner and outer actions, most of which one can do only for oneself.

1. Reinforce your identity separate from the patient's.
2. Always move from your center, not the patient's.

3. Tap into your unused, unlimited inner strengths and creative resources.
4. Continually acknowledge all feelings, positive and negative.
5. Get information and get help.
6. Work out your own plan for surviving whole.
7. Be responsible and take control.
8. Accept what you cannot change.
9. Eliminate the words "blame" and "excuse" from your vocabulary.
10. Make no promises about the future.
11. Face and explore the worst possible events in your future.
12. Use respite services regularly for extended blocks of time.
13. Develop an emotional detachment from your caregiving tasks.
14. Train yourself to be proactive rather than reactive.
15. Enjoy humor regularly; it assists the immune system.
16. Get a support system that works for you.
17. Be flexible, willing to learn a new thing—a new way.
18. Regroove your brain with positive reinforcement.
19. Develop an exercise regimen of both kinds, body and soul.
20. Look for small joys.

These strategies are a conscious and integrated part of my caregiving. As I stated earlier, caregiving is a learning process. New caregivers are a lot like new parents, learning as we go along. Often when acquaintances ask me how I am doing with Hughes, I tell them it is a learning experience—like being in a school that requires the strictest personal discipline. I believe caregivers are pioneers in understanding human behavior that is not yet in textbooks.

The best caregiving is individualized and tailored to the needs and strengths of the patient. One of the federal regulations for long-term care facilities is that each facility must develop a comprehensive care plan for each resident. In OSCAR Report 18, one-fourth of both SNF and NF failed to comply with this regulation.

Of course, it is a lot easier to give personalized care in the home. But whether in the home or in an institution, the primary caregiver will need to develop coping strategies for surviving the emotional stresses involved. Since each caregiver is unique, each necessarily determines the order of the strategies; this is mine. Also, of course, they overlap: several strategies will be working at one time.

1. *Reinforce your identity separate from the patient's.* While Hughes and I were very much a couple and a team, we were still two distinct individuals.

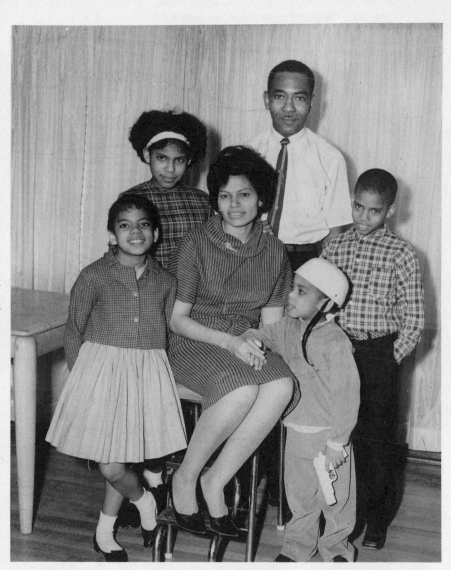

1. The Shanks family, 1962, Kansas City. Lela (seated); clockwise from lower left: Shela, Nena, Hughes, Cedric, Eric.

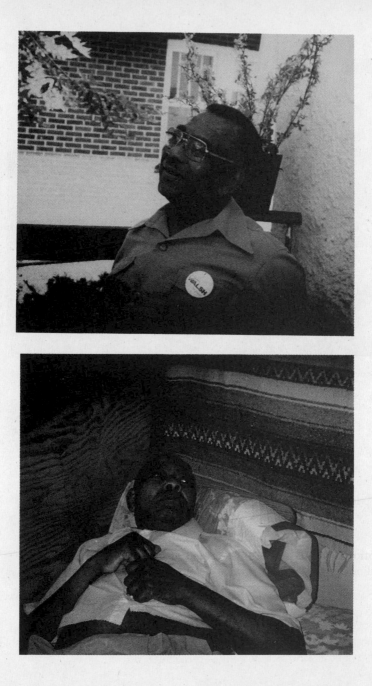

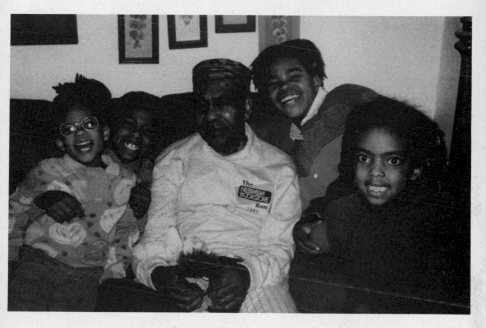

2. (top left) Hughes in 1982, just before the onset of AD. At this time he was actively involved in political campaigning. Photo by Dean Achen.

3. (bottom left) Hughes waking from a night's sleep, 1994. His shirt is cut at the waistline and there is a plastic cover on the pillow for reasons of hygiene. Note also the partition Cedric erected to enable Hughes to find the bathroom.

4. (above) Hughes with Shela's children, 1994. From left to right, Orchid, Zenith, Hughes, Orpheus, and Zoë. Hughes is wearing his t-shirt from the 1994 Nebraska Bookstore Run, in which he walked three miles.

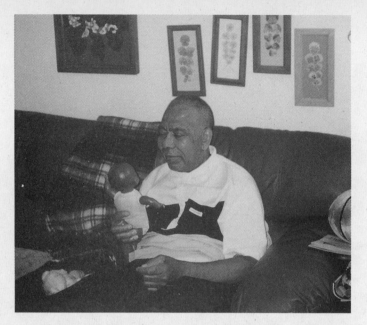

5. Hughes with a doll, November 1995.

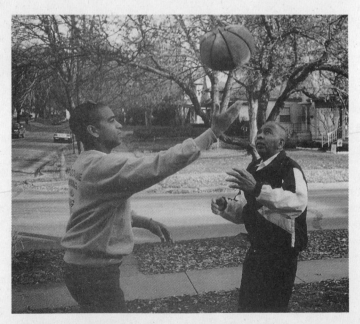

6. Eric and Hughes playing ball, November 1995.

When he got AD, I had known for many years that his life was not my life. I also knew that only I could validate myself. But I had not known this in the first half of our marriage. In those years I had not yet consciously discovered my own inner being, the center of my life. I did not yet know what it meant to be alive.

As a young homemaker I remember saying dramatically, "My children are my life," "My family is my life," "My husband is my life." In fact, in those years I felt I could not exist without Hughes. I depended upon what he did and what my relationship with him was from moment to moment for my happiness and for defining my existence. I was constantly trying to change and control Hughes. (That was twenty-five years before Melody Beattie's book made "codependent" a household word.)[3] It was not until I received help from the sisters that I learned to experience a level of awareness that makes one's life feel whole and complete within itself. I also began to understand and accept that each of us is responsible for creating his or her own happiness because happiness comes from within—another reason for rejecting the dismal picture of my future painted by Hughes's diagnosticians.

In order to bolster and reinforce my separate identity, immediately after Hughes's diagnosis I held conversations with myself to reaffirm my life and my existence: "You still have your life. This is your life within you. . . . You get to decide whether you are going to be miserable or not. . . . You do not have AD. Hughes has AD . . . . Apparently, you need this job of caregiving for your inner training. . . . There is still a way for you to take care of Hughes and live your life to the fullest. No, you do not know right now how it is possible for all of that to work out. You do not have to know. Take one step at a time. The way will open. Anything is possible. All you have to do is get through this moment. . . . Hughes's having AD does not have to be bad for you. You have a choice. . . . This is happening to you for a good purpose. Go with the flow. . . . Work on your anger and rage. You can grow from this." Over and over again I held these conversations with myself.

I was fortunate that when Hughes developed AD, I was in a period of great enthusiasm about living my own life. I had reached age sixty in 1987, and that was like crossing the Rubicon, since my mother had died at fifty-four. I felt as if I had been given a new lease on life. Every new day was a bonus. I knew the joy that comes from just being alive. I felt whole and complete, and nothing, including AD, could take that away from me.

2. *Always move from your center, not the patient's.* I usually use prayer to center. To center means to be aware of one's existence in that moment. It

is the basic awareness and acknowledgment of the life within us. Our center is at the core of our being. The patient's center is at the core of her or his being. Moving from our center puts us in touch with the Source of Life, and it is here that we find the meaning and the purpose for everything that happens in our lives, including AD. Only the individual can find his or her center.

When I was a codependent with Hughes, I did not know what it meant to have my own center or how to become centered. It is true that I had grown up in a Christian church, but I never recall hearing that I had an inner life that connected me to the Source of Life. Neither do I recall hearing that my inner life would always be there with me for as long as I lived, and that no one could ever get to it or take it away from me. I knew intellectually that every human being has a soul or an inner spirit, but I knew nothing about my own on a conscious, everyday level. I certainly knew nothing about the urgency of my need to practice the development and nourishment of my inner life. I depended upon being with Hughes for my very existence. I thought I could not live without him.

Since men usually made their jobs their center, it was common for women of my generation to believe that our spouses should be the center of our lives. Yet I often felt miserable and empty and did not know why. I did not understand that feelings of emptiness are natural consequences when we substitute another's life for our own. Our inner being remains stunted and undeveloped when we try to live through others.

Once I had learned to move from my center, I made the connection between my faith and my daily life. In fact, it is the act of centering that anchors us in and to our faith. There we find the inner strength to transcend outer circumstances, including the life changes and the devastation wrought by AD.

3. *Tap into your unused, unlimited inner strengths and creative resources.* Once I began to move from my center and to connect with the Source of Life, I discovered that creativity, inner strength, and solutions to problems are infinite; indeed, the solutions are often simple and uncomplicated. The only limits on our inner resources are those we impose on ourselves. The potential for developing our strengths has been with us since birth, but each of us has to learn to access them from the inside out.

I knew from my mother's life that one could be strong and creative, but Mama never talked about how she did it. She just did it. Strength and creativity seemed as natural to her as breathing, and I took everything about her for granted. It never occurred to me to ask my mother about her faith and where her strength came from. I wonder how many grown children ever have such conversations with their parents. At the time, I was deeply involved in going through the outer motions and appearances of living a religious life without knowing that what I needed had to be on the inside. It was from the sisters that I learned how to activate my own strengths and creativity through the conscious development of my inner life. I also learned what a mistake it is ever to take anyone or anything for granted.

A caregiver needs many inner strengths, including (but not limited to) patience, determination, faith, perseverance, courage, and hope. When I was a young mother, I remember saying, as if it were something to be proud of, "Oh, I don't have any patience!" Since Hughes has had AD, I have had to become a close companion of patience, and still I am impatient.

Patience is the capacity or habit of enduring adversity or pain with fortitude. We feel this pain from within whenever we are unable to have our own way in the moment that we want it. When we tell an AD patient (or anyone else, for that matter) to do something, we often want it to be done now. But AD patients do not always understand "right now"; AD patients require time. By definition they are "patients," and we do "wait on them." Waiting is intrinsic to patience, and it is the waiting and the enduring that causes us inner pain and suffering. But theologian Paul Tillich says, "To endure the pain is more horrible and more difficult than anything else in the world. And yet, to endure it is the only way by which we can attain to the ultimate meaning, joy, and freedom in our lives."[4] The patience of caregivers makes every day a miracle for Hughes, because it is through the patience of others at home and at day care that he is still able to enjoy some quality in his life, even as a person with dementia.

Caregivers also have to have a lot of courage. Courage is defined as the firmness of spirit that faces danger or extreme difficulty without flinching or retreating. It is mind-boggling to think that we are born with the potential for all the courage we need in our lives. It is right here on the inside of ourselves, ours for the taking.

All of us show courage every day, often taking it for granted. But taking things for granted is like sleepwalking through life. When we tap into our inner strengths, we have to do so consciously, give our attention to it. As caregivers, it takes courage to face our fears of the future, look them in the eye, and eliminate them one by one. It takes courage to put our loved ones in adult day care, and probably even more courage when the time comes to place them in a nursing home. It takes courage to persevere and to endure daily. It takes lots of courage to break through our pride and to ask for help.

It takes courage to give up our loved ones as we knew them in the past and to begin a new and fulfilling life with them as they are now.

In my years with the sisters, whenever I despaired or complained about anything to them, they told me, "Discouragement is the anesthetic that the devil uses when he is getting ready to cut your heart out." They taught me never to give in to discouragement.

4. *Continually acknowledge all feelings, positive and negative.* Because we are not volunteers for this new and difficult job, beginning caregivers often experience a concentrated excess of hostile emotions—from anger to hate to resentment to rage to bitterness to self-pity to embarrassment to fear. We may run the gamut of all of our negative feelings in one moment.

In addition to learning to acknowledge my negative feelings, I also learned to express them verbally, especially my anger, when that seemed necessary. The sisters taught me that anger is one of the many forms of energy and most often defines our hostile and negative feelings; they taught me to use meditations and prayers as the conduit for constructively channeling the energy from my anger. Sometimes I bellow out a prayer of thanksgiving for the difficulty of that moment or break out into a hymn—this is a way of making angry energy work positively. The sisters said this was a way of accommodating our hate, as opposed to multiplying it by projecting it onto others. It was a technique that had helped me through the most difficult times of child rearing, when our four children in turn became hostile and rebellious teenagers. But when Hughes got AD, I found myself acknowledging and expressing my anger nonstop. There are so many startling changes that the new caregiver must process and deal with simultaneously. The patient is in and out of lucidity; the caregiver is still hanging on to the lucid moments, not wanting to give them up; the patient is deteriorating and creating new problems faster than the caregiver knows how to handle them; the caregiver is having to take on more and more of the patient's chores. I did not like any of this. I was not just exhausted from the extra load of physical work; I was exhausted from feeling angry.

I started reading everything I could find on anger, rage, and hostility. I began to remember how the sisters had talked about "nonresistance" and "going with the flow of life." The writer Clyde Reid tells us, "Lean into your pain."[5] But now that Hughes had AD, the pain and the flow came in such intensity and volume that it felt like a flood. I began to wonder: Was there a dimension of consciousness or being beyond repression or the need for expression of anger? Was there an alternative to anger?

In the 1960s the last word on anger had been that we harmed our bodies if we kept it bottled up inside ourselves. We were advised to express our true feelings, always. We were told in the vernacular of those days to "let it all hang out." But that advice was beginning to seem obsolete to me.

In researching anger I discussed "going with the flow" with Chris Milne, Hughes's psychologist at the Veterans Administration. One study said that hostility could hurt your heart.[6] Another concluded that anger is a poison to the body: according to Dr. Redford Williams, a professor of psychiatry at Duke University Medical Center in Durham, North Carolina, "It isn't the impatience, the ambition or the work drive. It's the anger: It sends your blood pressure skyrocketing. It provokes your body to create unhealthy chemicals." All of this frightened me, since in the beginning stages I was angry so much of the time. But Dr. Williams went on to say, "Avoid *feeling* angry in the first place, and you won't need to suppress your anger."[7] This was what I needed to work on.

I observed that the crucial time for me to "avoid anger" when working with Hughes was in that initial moment when he refused to cooperate (most likely because he did not understand; after all, he is demented). I continue to find that when I accept him as he is and "lean into the pain," my anger is mitigated. When this happens, it is as if I become a part of the Alzheimer's and it becomes a part of me. In those too rare times, Hughes and I work together inseparably for his care. This was the new dimension of awareness I was looking for: avoiding anger in the first place. I am finding that this takes a lot of discipline and practice and is a lifelong process.

In order to reinforce positive feelings, I learned from the sisters to use meditation, contemplation, singing, and deep breathing and—most important—to spend my thoughts on praise and thankfulness for my life. They once told me that if I started a list of what I had to be thankful for, it would extend for miles and still be incomplete. Prayer, like anger, is also a form of energy. As French surgeon and 1912 Nobel Prize winner Alexis Carrel wrote, "Prayer is the most powerful form of energy that we can generate."[8] Our thoughts and minds make us who and what we are. It is in our thoughts that we create our own nervous tension and our own emotional stresses.

The sisters recommended early morning meditation before beginning one's day. I have found that this can be done only through the use of force on the self. A. J. Russell, in his book *God at Eventide*, says that "the violence we should use in life is that of discipline and self-conquest."[9] It is in a meditative and contemplative state that our minds are emptied and creativity flows.

5. *Get information and get help.* After Hughes's second diagnosis in 1988,

I needed new information relating to every aspect of our lives. Our old way of life was gone, and I would have to learn a new way to live. First, I wanted to know everything about this disease. Why did Hughes not know me and our children? Why did he not recognize his home of thirty years? Why did he hide things? Why was he paranoid? Why did he make ridiculous accusations? Why did he pat dogs that were not there? I knew the truth of the cliché "Knowledge is the key to understanding." I had endless questions about the disease and how I would manage Hughes in our home.

I read all the books and articles I could find on AD in our libraries. The number of books was limited, but there were countless articles in gerontology and geriatric journals and magazines. The more I read about the disease, the better I understood why Hughes acted as he did; this helped to relieve some of my anger and resentment. Also, learning about the stages of AD and what I could expect in the future eased some of my fears and anxieties. I learned a lot from the Alzheimer's Association newsletter and monthly meetings as well.

In addition to information about the disease, I needed legal information. I immediately got a durable power of attorney, which permits me to act on Hughes's behalf. But I had other questions. Should I make changes in names on bank accounts, titles to our home and car, safety deposit box, and any other joint financial matters? Legal advice allows caregivers to make intelligent decisions and reduces stress.

Further, I needed information on nursing homes in case I should have to institutionalize Hughes. I decided to visit several nursing homes within a thirty-mile radius of our home. Friends volunteered to visit them with me, but I felt this was a job I should do alone. Some of the homes were clean and odor free (among them, interestingly, some of the least expensive); others were not. In 1989, monthly costs ranged from $1,400 to $3,000. At that time our income would have covered the $1,400 facility, but that would have left very little for me to live on. I filled out applications for Hughes at three of these nursing homes, and I keep up his registration at one of them by calling and renewing it every three months; the other two call me periodically for an update. (See chapter 10 for differences among nursing homes for AD patients.)

After getting information on costs, I contacted the Veterans Administration and my state's Department of Social Services to find out what help would be available if I had to put Hughes in a nursing home. I could pay for a few months out of our savings, but once they were gone, could Hughes qualify for Medicaid, the state-administered welfare program? A representative of the Department of Social Services informed me that every state had a Spousal Impoverishment Program, which was mandated by Congress in 1988 as a part of the Catastrophic Coverage Act. Under that program the well spouse no longer had to sell the family home or go bankrupt before the disabled spouse could qualify for assistance with nursing home costs. (I know one woman who divorced her husband who had AD so that he could qualify for Medicaid.) In some states the well spouse could keep half the combined value of all the couple's countable resources up to $70,740.[10] Further, if the total of all of the couple's combined countable resources was $14,148 or less, the well spouse could keep it all. I also learned about Medicaid's Services Waivers for the Elderly, a program that assists aged persons like Hughes to remain in their own homes (see the last section in chapter 9).[11] Caregivers can contact their own state's social services department for information on these or similar programs.

I asked the Veterans Administration what help might be available to Hughes if I had to put him in a home. I learned that the VA officer of the county in which the veteran lives is the person to contact for information on VA nursing home services.

I visited the Nebraska Department of Health and read the evaluation reports from the latest state inspections of all of the nursing homes I had visited. These reports are public information. Caregivers cannot afford to be timid. Caregivers have to ask questions. Caregivers have to investigate.

I further learned that each state had an ombudsman program to serve as "the 'voice' of the residents" in nursing homes.[12] Families with a loved one in a nursing home were no longer alone with their unresolved complaints. They could contact the state office building or their state department on aging and ask for the Long-Term-Care Ombudsman Program—evidence of the growing interest and determination to improve living conditions in our country's nursing homes.

Assembling all this information greatly relieved my fears and anxieties about our future. Now I could concentrate on creating a new life for Hughes and for me. But the more I learned, the more I realized that I needed all the help I could get.

6. *Work out your own plan for surviving whole.* After getting information, the caregiver is able to make decisions about her or his future. Each caregiver is different—just as each patient is—and therefore each person's plan will be made with that uniqueness in mind. The main goal of my plan was to provide the best care possible for Hughes, preferably in our home, at the same time taking care of myself and living my life completely.

In summary, my plan included taking legal steps for my financial protection; physically restructuring our home for Hughes's needs; putting Hughes in day care; cultivating a pool of friends and paid sitters for respite (see chapter 9); registering Hughes at nursing homes; getting mental health help for both of us from the VA; going back to work to supplement our income; and allowing time to care for myself.

7. *Be responsible and take control.* After the patient has been diagnosed as having AD, caregivers can relieve themselves of a lot of stress and anxiety by taking charge and making decisions about the future for the patient. Of course, taking control is a formidable task for many of us; in fact, it can be downright scary. But when AD sets in and the patient is no longer able to live alone and care for him- or herself, someone has to step in and be responsible.

Sometimes the well spouse, for whatever reason, is unable to take charge, and responsibility for the AD patient falls on the grown children. Indeed, sometimes both parents need care. It can be very difficult for the grown child of an AD patient to assume the position overnight of giving directions to a parent and making important decisions about the parent's future and life. This is difficult at any age. Some people think of it as role reversal, but I do not. I believe it should be a natural part of our maturation and evolution to form adult relationships with our parents, whatever their mental capabilities.

There are also many well spouses who have difficulty taking charge of the patient. Some caregivers, both men and women, have said to me of their AD spouses, "She doesn't like going to day care," or "She won't go," or "He does not like it when I leave him with a sitter," or "He won't let me have time off." But I believe these statements come out of our denial, because if we really accept that our loved ones are now demented, we no longer look to them for decision-making. Just as we would not permit a three-year-old to make family choices, neither can we permit a demented spouse or parent to do so. Once we take charge and start making the necessary decisions, we begin to see how we can get on with our new life.

8. *Accept what you cannot change.* The writer Katherine Mansfield has said, "I find that when I accept a thing, it undergoes a change."[13] Likewise, when AD caregivers accept the reality of the disease, we see solutions to daily problems more clearly. Nonacceptance is like banging one's head against a wall.

I found that when I gave Hughes up as my husband and as the man I once knew, I was then able to meet him on a deeper level—one closer to his heart and his soul. Acceptance permits communication without verbal or physical cues. It is as if a process of mental osmosis takes over. Hughes knows when he is being accepted and when he is being rejected. A family friend of many years visited us when Hughes was well into the second stage of the disease. I had tried to prepare her for his condition, but she would not accept that Hughes no longer recognized her, even though he refused to stay in the same room with her. Today when someone who visits in our home is accepting of him, he always gives that person his doll or his paper or a ball or other token.

It is our nonacceptance of a present reality that feeds into depression and self-pity. The sisters called self-pity "preserved hate," whereas self-awareness is the key to acceptance.

9. *Eliminate the words "blame" and "excuse" from your vocabulary.* It is not unusual to blame the patient for being ill, especially when the illness causes great inconvenience to us. Blame gives us a sadistic kind of satisfaction and shifts our pain onto someone else. But in blaming others, I abdicate responsibility for what I should be doing in that moment in my own life. Blaming can only speak to events that are past, dead, and irretrievable. It closes us off from our creative center and the solutions we need to solve the problems. In blaming, we are like puppets on someone else's string, since it is impossible to blame someone else and take responsibility at the same time. When I catch myself blaming Hughes (or anyone), I try to hurry to my center, where I find the inner strength to accept responsibility for my life in that moment.

Excuses are the natural children of blame. One day I was stunned to realize that I could not use Hughes's AD as an excuse for my behavior or for anything. I had learned from the sisters, who quoted Sigmund Freud, that "there are no excuses." I thought I had accepted this, and I had tried to teach the concept to our children. But every day brings its own challenge, and the life skills I thought I had learned were being tested daily, Hughes's illness being such a convenient and acceptable excuse. I found that there was no going back for me to a former life filled with blame, codependency, and excuses. I had to affirm my existence by accepting the responsibility for my life, including my pain.

10. *Make no promises about the future.* Some parents and spouses before the onset of an illness will try to cajole family members into making promises such as "Promise me you will never put me in a nursing home" or as Hughes told me many years before AD, "I don't want you to become burdened with me if I get so I can't take care of myself. Put me in a nursing

home" (he also requested that no machines be used to keep him alive). Either way, this is manipulation and should be seen as such. No one can manipulate us without our permission.

If patients in the early stage of AD try to extract a promise of continued in-home care, there are several responses open to the caregiver who remembers that one cannot reason with dementia: reassuring our loved one that "I am going to do the very best for you that I can do. I love you"; distracting the person from such thoughts, according to the patient's level of cognition; validating the person's concern and feeling for him- or herself at that moment, without actually making a promise. Combining all three responses might also be workable. Some caregivers even lie effectively when they determine that is what it will take at that moment to give comfort and relief to their loved one. Such untruths have been referred to as "therapeutic lies."[14]

Making promises about the unknown, even in good conscience, entraps us and causes untold anxieties and stress. Keeping all our options open frees us to be creative about solutions to future problems and reduces stress.

11. *Face and explore the worst possible events in your future.* When a loved one is ill, we sometimes live in fear of the future. But the way to overcome a fear is to face it. Walk right into it. Look it in the eye. The inner strength we need is always right there inside us if we will use it.

We can make a list of the worst things that could happen: being left alone, the institutionalization or death of our loved one, bankruptcy, or whatever we fear. Discuss all these possibilities and fears with family, close friends, a counselor, lawyer, doctor. If you worry about nursing home costs, go to your state's social services department and the VA (if applicable). Do not let foolish pride stand in your way. Few of us have enough savings to pay extended nursing home costs, but it is self-destructive to complain or worry without looking for solutions. Solutions are infinite. Good preparations now can help negate future guilt.

An example of my earliest fears involved what Hughes might do to me after I had moved out of our bedroom. I was worried that one night I might wake up and find him attacking me, since he often thought I was an impostor in those early years. It came to me to put up barricades every night by stacking dining room chairs and boards in my bedroom doors. Since I am a light sleeper, I felt that those obstructions would give me the warning I needed if he ever tried to come in while I slept. Occasionally, he would come and look over the barricades, and sometimes he seemed puzzled, but he never tried to force his way in or attack me.

12. *Use respite services regularly for extended blocks of time.* Studies show that respite—having someone else step in and take over the caregiver's duties—is the overall greatest need of caregivers. For that period, of whatever length, the caregiver is free from the mental and physical pressures of the patient's constant need for care.

Respite care has been my survival lifeline. No one in our society works twenty-four hours around the clock, day in and day out nonstop, without being relieved. Yet that is precisely what the caregiver of an AD patient has to do. I have often heard speakers (who had never been hands-on caregivers) encourage others to volunteer for a couple of hours when possible to relieve the caregivers. I always want to scream when I hear that! Of course, two hours is better than nothing and greatly appreciated, but in order to continue on twenty-four-hour duty, caregivers need much more than an occasional two hours' relief. They need larger blocks of time—four hours at a minimum—on a dependable weekly schedule. To achieve such a schedule, the caregiver has to be creative, determined, and persistent in finding ways of getting relief.

Chapter 9 discusses the different sources a caregiver can explore for respite services, some more available in urban than in rural areas.

13. *Develop an emotional detachment from your caregiving tasks.* The primary caregiver cannot retain the same familiar relationship with the patient as in the past. Because we have to live with the patient as she or he is today, a new relationship must be formed. Carrying the emotions of our past relationship with the patient into the present dissipates our energy and weighs us down. It is natural that there will be a period of ambiguity and ambivalence, especially when the patient still has some moments of lucidity, so detachment will take time. It will not happen all at once, for caregiving is an evolutionary process. But acceptance of the reality makes emotional detachment possible. Our daughter Nena once said, after talking to her dad on the phone, "It's like having another little brother."

Emotional detachment also releases us from interpreting everything our loved one says and does as a personal attack on us, and thereby relieves us of some self-pity and blame. Several steps were helpful to me over time. For example, when Hughes made accusations, I reminded myself that the dementia was talking, since the husband I once knew was now gone. Further, I stopped looking to Hughes to give me something back in our relationship; this made my caregiving tasks more routine and businesslike. I also stopped trying to hang on to his lucid moments, since they took me back to what used to be.

One caregiver states that through detachment she is able to treat the tasks involved in her husband's care matter-of-factly, as if she is working on a job.

14. *Train yourself to be proactive rather than reactive.* When we simply react, we put ourselves on the defensive and permit others to determine our ground rules. But we can be proactive, determining those ground rules in advance. Each of us has his or her own mind. The one power over which we have full control is our free will. It is up to each of us alone to determine how to act, how to feel, and how to use our energies, regardless of the outer circumstances in our lives.

An AD patient may do or say anything, especially to the primary caregiver, at any time. When Hughes was in the accusatory phase, I multiplied the stress when I tried to defend myself against his bizarre charges. For example, in the beginning, when he said I was out with "my boyfriend," I would get so angry! But in reacting to him, I was permitting a person who no longer had the use of his mind to determine my mood, my course of action, and my life. We abdicate control of our own existence when we merely react to others.

When we get back to our center, our inner life, we stop reacting to people and to events. In this way, we affirm our identity as a human being.

15. *Enjoy humor regularly; it assists the immune system.* Some caregivers see no humor in their lives or their patients' lives. Yet even though a loved one may be chronically or incurably ill, this does not dictate that all of life must be sad and forlorn for the caregiver and the patient. Life is not a one-dimensional thing; it has many facets, with caregiving and illness and death only parts of the whole. As we expand our consciousness, we are able to grow and enjoy the fullness of life, especially the humor.

The late journalist Norman Cousins recounted in his book *Anatomy of an Illness* how laughter helped him overcome three life-threatening ailments. He called a hearty laugh "internal jogging."[15] In *Head First,* Cousins presented research evidence from studies conducted at the UCLA School of Medicine that laughter increases the immune cells, or T-cells, which help us fight off infections and cancers; by the same token, anger, hostility, depression, dejection, and other negative emotions suppress the immune system. Cousins quotes Dr. James Walsh, who said over fifty years ago, "Laughter brushes aside the worries and fears that set the stage for sickness."[16] Stop to think: Isn't it difficult to be mad or sad or dejected and to laugh at the same time?

There have been numerous funny incidents in our lives since Hughes has had AD. One night about five years ago after I had tucked him in bed and was leaving the room, he said, "There is something flying around out there, and those eyes are looking in here at me." This was during Hughes's hallucinating phase, when he saw dogs and cats and babies that were not there. I was very tired that night, and all I wanted to do was go to my room and fall on the bed. So, quickly trying to think of something reassuring, I turned to him and said, "Oh, honey, there is nothing flying around out there. Those are just the eyes of God looking in on you. Now you don't mind the eyes of God watching you, do you?" With his own big eyes looking very sure of himself, he said, "Well, there is still something flying around out there and looking in here at me." I patted him, hurriedly, and left the room.

Later that night I was relaxing and reading when suddenly I thought I saw something fly by in the next room. I did a double take but quickly scolded myself: "Now, girl, get yourself together! One of you in this family has to keep some sense!" I went back to my book, but once again I thought I saw something fly by. I got up and looked. It was a bat! My first thought, though I had read that bats were usually harmless, was to be sure Hughes was safe. I hastily closed all the doors to his room and opened the door to the basement. Using newspaper, I swished the bat down there. Then I called Animal Control, and within thirty minutes the bat was gone. Hughes had been right after all. There *were* eyes out there looking in at him.

Humorous things often happen when we take our walks. One day as we were walking to the day-care center, it was rainy and very muddy. Hughes is not quite as agile at seventy-five as he once was, and sometimes he jumps over mud into other mud. This particular morning, by the time we arrived at the center, he had mud up to his ankle on one shoe and on both pants legs. I had tried to wipe some of it off with the few tissues I had but ended up getting it on me. We looked a mess! When the day-care staff saw us, they burst into laughter, and we all had a good chuckle.

Another time when we were walking in the rain, I was carrying the umbrella over both of us. After a few blocks, Hughes acted as if he wanted to hold the umbrella, so I let him have it. He immediately put it only over himself.

Once when I was helping Hughes wash his hands, he started washing mine. I said, "No not mine!" Suddenly, he seemed to understand; he laughed and said, "That's a goody." Then he turned to me and asked, "What world is this?" I told him we were on the planet earth. I could have cried about his question, but I decided to laugh instead. As caregivers, we have a choice. We can let the continuous drone of our loved one overwhelm us, or we can find the humor and release our stress.

When I first started attending the meetings of the local Alzheimer's Association, the president always had as a part of the program a time when everyone could share funny stories related to caregiving. She once told about her mother-in-law, who hummed or sang continually. The president called the tune the Alzheimer's National Anthem.

Sandy Bliss, Alzheimer's program manager at the day-care center, tells a story about a male patient who played a harmonica all the time. One day when he was out in the courtyard, Sandy looked up and saw that he had climbed the big apple tree and was hanging by his knees, playing his harmonica upside down. Sandy says, "That's when we cut the apple tree down."

The funniest story I have heard was told by my friend Norma, who took care of her husband, Gordon, in their home for over ten years before his death. One of her coping strategies was to take him for long car trips, which he loved. But once, as they were returning home, he criticized her driving relentlessly all the way back to town. When they reached home, she scolded him in turn and went into the house. He sat in the car for a while. Finally, he came in and announced, "I fired that driver for insubordination."

16. *Get a support system that works for you.* Caregivers need all the help and support they can get. It is foolish to try to go it alone. No matter how strong we might feel, we are still imperfect, interdependent beings. The creation of a strong and dependable support system is essential to any plan for survival. Persons who have a positive outlook on life provide the best support system. Negative people, whether family members or friends, sap our energies and give us nothing in return. When Hughes was in the beginning stage, I avoided complainers and negative people like the plague. When I returned from visiting Shela and her family in 1993, the most prevalent remark made to me was, "Isn't it too bad you couldn't stay but four days?" But the positive people gave me great support by saying, "I am so glad you got to visit Shela and her family!"

It is natural for caregivers to look to family members as their primary source of support; that is one of the purposes of a family—to provide a built-in base. Typically, the well spouse of a person diagnosed with AD first turns to the children; if the patient is widowed, the siblings usually turn to one another. I learned quickly, however, that it is best to use someone who is less emotionally involved with the patient as a sounding board. Our children were too distressed; they needed their own sounding boards to help them deal with their anger and rage. They were in no shape emotionally to handle my dumping on them. Once I stopped, they felt a freedom to ask questions about their dad and offer solace in their own time.

Our daughter-in-law Chris, in Oregon, was my sounding board in the hardest times of those early years. When I talked about Hughes's mental deterioration with Chris, she did not feel as threatened as our own children; Hughes was not her father. She called several times each week so I could talk about my feelings. Being honest is essential to coping.

Chris and I sometimes had a contest between us. She was working on improving her relationship with her own two children, and of course I was working on improving my relationship with Hughes. Using a scale of one to ten, we rated both our angry feelings and our behavior for each day during several weeks. We kept notes, and at the end of each week we tallied our scores and discussed our mistakes and what we could do differently the next time. The winner received an imaginary star. We laughed at ourselves, but that exercise with Chris and our long talks were great stress releasers and helped me through my most difficult days.

The support Hughes and I have received from our children, relatives, and friends has been extraordinary. Each individual contributes in her or his own way from whatever inner resources each has. Though the greatest need of the caregiver is respite service, not every member of our support system is physically, mentally, or emotionally equipped to provide personal hands-on care. Just as not everyone is proficient at mathematics, not everyone is adept at caregiving. We cannot give what we do not have, but one who cares about the patient and the caregiver can always do something—and we have received a variety of unusual and unexpected kinds of support. For example, when Hughes was in the beginning stage of the disease, his friend Dean volunteered to screen in our front porch; he and his wife, Sonja, thought Hughes might better enjoy sitting there if it was made private. Little did I know then how much this locked, screened porch would help me years later as a safe and secure area where Hughes could walk or sit while I worked nearby at my computer.

It is not uncommon for family and friends to rally around the patient and the caregiver in the early stages. But as the years go by and the patient's mentality continues to deteriorate, it is difficult for others to sustain the same level of support. They grow accustomed to seeing the primary caregiver do most or all of the work, and of course they are all involved with their own lives and their own daily hassles and problems. The smart caregiver has to be prepared for those times when she or he must go it alone, including holidays and periods of the caregiver's illness. This is why it is so important to develop a pool of paid sitters of all ages.

In addition to my family and friends, support groups have been an important part of my support system. These groups usually form out of the

Alzheimer's Association, adult day-care centers, state departments on aging, nursing homes, and churches. A few large employers are also beginning to encourage the formation of on-site caregiver support groups. Small groups typically have a loose structure with a primary objective of allowing members to express feelings. This opportunity to vent is a must for beginning caregivers, who are probably traumatized and in shock for months after their loved one's diagnosis. When AD support groups first formed, very little was known about the disease and patient management; neither were there AD day-care centers. Today, however, we know more about the disease and can now expand our vision of support groups to include not only a place for venting feelings but also a place for role-playing solutions and for discovering new techniques of patient management.

In addition, nursing home caregivers and in-home caregivers have different concerns and problems, and it is important for support groups to recognize these differences in order to meet the needs of both. And since neither category is monolithic—one caregiver's patient is in the beginning stage, another's in the middle stage, and still another's in the terminal stage— it is helpful for large support groups to have trained facilitators and structured assistance for caregivers facing any of the three stages. The knowledge of such a structure might say to the new caregiver that given time, one can move from the initial stage of constant rage and anger and self-pity, and go on to problem solving. One of the greatest stress reducers for me is to solve whatever the current problem is in Hughes's care.

17. *Be flexible, willing to learn a new thing—a new way.* As caregivers we must learn to accommodate a new and greater level of physical and mental work. Sometimes I say I feel like a rubber band, stretched and pulled this way and that. Life is ever fluid, ever changing. And the marvelous quality about us as human beings is our ability to adapt, to learn, to grow, and to change at any age. It may be true that old dogs can't learn new tricks, but old people can.[17]

It is our flexibility that permits us to make the ongoing changes in our life-style necessary to accommodate the AD patient. It is flexibility that enables us to "lean into the pain" and to go with the flow. Adaptation permits our bodies to shift gears and change schedules in order to meet the erratic demands of caregiving. For instance, I never have any problem going right back to sleep, no matter how many times I may have to get up with Hughes. The more numerous the interruptions, the more valued the remaining sleep. It is as if our bodies have a stability that is always in flux, since our internal clock can be set and reset again and again.

Rigidity is the opposite of flexibility. It is difficult to say which causes us the greatest pain, the added work load of caring for the patient or our rigidity. But flexibility and willingness to learn enable us to develop our unfulfilled selves even as caregivers. Hughes's illness has forced me to discover a whole new part of myself I never knew existed. It is as if he had to become incapacitated in order for me to grow in unknown and unexplored areas of self-realization.

Hughes was a fixer. He fixed everything; all I had to do was complain. Now I have become a fixer, doing everything from replacing door locks to hauling 400 pounds of dirt and putting in a lawn. I had not used a spade in decades, and it was such hard work that I had to turn over and plant the yard in sections. It took me a couple of weeks, so that as the grass came up some stood one inch, some two inches, some three. But it all came up! What a joy to peek out each day at the crack of dawn and see a green back yard that I had started from scratch! It had never occurred to me that we could develop muscles in our sixties. Now I know we can develop muscles well into our eighties if we exercise. This experience gave me a new sense of accomplishment and self-confidence.

Flexibility also releases us from always trying to be in control, always insisting on our way or no way. Some helper groups advocate that their approach should be the only approach. But flexibility teaches us that the ways of approaching and solving the daily problems we face are infinite. Just as our muscles increase in size to accommodate heavier weights, our minds can expand in breadth and depth to accommodate our ever widening world. Given flexibility, there is no limit to creation.

18. *Regroove your brain with positive reinforcement.* Our thoughts, both conscious and unconscious, control us. We are what we give our thoughts and minds to. It is in our thoughts, often the unconscious ones, that our behavior originates. It is always our own negative thoughts that defeat us; no one else resides inside our brains.

The process of regrooving the brain begins with becoming conscious. As we become conscious, we are then able to step outside ourselves and watch the constant litany of our negativity.[18] After the deed is done, how many times have we asked ourselves, "Why did I say that? Why did I do that?" It is as if we were programmed from birth to respond negatively to people and to events in our lives. That is why throughout human history the sages have advised us to develop a regimen of meditation, prayer, contemplation, chanting to assist us (or rescue us) in controlling our thoughts and minds.[19] The writer A. B. Simpson states that "the only way to be armed against them [negative thoughts] is to refuse them and the source from which they come."[20]

In crisis incidents with Hughes, my most immediate help is in forcing myself to repeat aloud short positive affirmations of belief: "This too will pass. There will be a way. I will be shown the answer. I will not be defeated. You can take it. Hang on. Hang tough." The trick is to use the force on oneself instead of on the patient.

Not until I met the sisters did I consciously learn how to acknowledge and appreciate that the creative and positive side of life is just as powerful and strong as the negative, if not stronger. Though I had seen my mother live creatively, I did not know how she did it. Of course, I knew intellectually that life had both a positive and a negative, but that knowledge had no conscious or practical application for me. Fritz Kunkel, psychologist and psychiatrist, explains in his book *Creation Continues* that the process of becoming a Christian is one of becoming fully conscious.[21] The Jewish writer Lawrence Kushner, in *Honey from the Rock,* says, "Eternal life is only awareness."[22] I learned from the sisters that through determination, perseverance, and self-discipline we can break the old habits and patterns of negative thoughts. It is possible to regroove our brains with positiveness.

19. *Develop an exercise regimen of both kinds, body and soul.* Physical exercise is probably my greatest stress reducer. My program includes walking, riding a stationary bicycle, and swimming. I walk four or five days, averaging a total of ten to twelve miles, each week. I also take Hughes for walks two to four times a week. In addition to parking our car a mile or more from the day-care center and walking the rest of the way, sometimes we walk in the morning before Eric takes his dad to day care; occasionally, we walk the entire two and a half miles to the center. Walks with Hughes are great adventures. I believe one of the reasons some AD patients become rigid and bedfast is that they never move. Hughes is now very sedentary and has to be prompted to stand up; he acts as if he no longer knows how. But once he is on his feet, he is a fast walker.

After I get Hughes safely into the day-care center, I feel as if I could fly. Aerobic exercise releases chemicals in the brain, called endorphins, which give us a natural high and boost our spirits. In 1994 my daughter-in-law Sherry and I walked thirteen miles in the Lincoln half-marathon, while Eric ran the twenty-six miles of the full marathon. I walked three hours and sixteen minutes. I cannot remember when I have had such a great time. I think my endorphins went wild! I was flabbergasted when an official of the Track Club came by afterward with a plaque stating that I had won first place for women of sixty-five plus. Also in 1994, Hughes and I walked in a three-mile road race completing the course in just under one hour. The officials said he was the oldest entrant. For the first two miles Hughes did fine, but for the last mile Kathleen (another walker and total stranger) and I—one on each side of Hughes—walked him to the finish line. What an experience!

Sharon, one of the sisters, told me that "exercise is to the body what prayer is to the soul." Today, medical science on a much larger scale than ever before acknowledges that what we do with our minds affects our bodies and our health. Norman Cousins was a pioneer in this area in our time; now, there are many books on that subject. Dr. Deepak Chopra's *Ageless Body, Timeless Mind,* for example, explains how the body and mind are inextricably connected.[23] Exercising both faith and the body can transform caregiving from a nightmare into a self-fulfilling experience.

20. *Look for small joys.* Joy, like patience and courage, faith and hope, is an inner strength that comes with us at birth. It is basic to life, and it is there in every age and stage of our lives. But like attitude, joy is a matter of our choice. It requires nothing of us except our acceptance. There is always plenty of it, and there is never a need to cancel or postpone it, since it is ever present in us. And though it is personal, it is impossible to hide. In its essence it is a form of praise and thanksgiving. My mother knew that joy even in her death.

Small joys are often the nonmaterialistic, unseen gifts all around us that we take for granted every day. The miraculous joy of waking up in the morning! (When I was a girl, I remember my father praying, "Thank You, Lord, for letting me wake up this morning while others passed in their slumber.") The joy of waking up without a headache or backache. The joy of being able to raise my hand to wash my own face. (I hurt my right elbow last spring, and for several weeks I could hardly lift my arm that high.) The joy of tenderly washing Hughes's face with a warm washcloth after I wake him up in the morning. The joy that comes from being able to walk. The joy of reaching home safely after driving in traffic. The connecting smile of a stranger. A kindness.

Alzheimer's program manager Sandy Bliss was once asked what she could find that was positive in caring for terminally ill patients who knew nothing. Sandy answered, "I can find joy in watching them smack their lips when I put ice cream in their mouths."

Caregiving forces us to fine-tune our values and our priorities. We learn to focus on what matters in life. The more conscious we become, the more we experience the joy of life that springs eternally out of the soul.

NINE

Finding Relief from Twenty-four-Hour Caregiving

It is my experience that in-home caregivers of long duration use a combination of respite services in order to survive. The several sources of help fall into two categories: fee-based services paid for by the caregiver, and services donated by others.

FEE-BASED SERVICES

AN ADULT DAY-CARE CENTER

In 1988 when Hughes began to need twenty-four-hour care, the most important step I took was to enroll him in an adult day-care center. I knew I had to have relief in order to keep going. I could no longer leave him home alone even for a short trip to the grocery store, and if I left him in the car while I ran an errand, he sometimes wandered off. Yet if I took him into the supermarket, the confusion overwhelmed him; often, he would not know me and would push the grocery cart as far away from me as possible. I had to follow him around in the store and wait until he knew who I was before he would leave with me. On one occasion, as I placed the grocery items on the check-out counter, Hughes put them one by one right back into the cart. He could no longer understand about putting them into bags; I waited to do that after I pushed the cart to the car. Clearly, the time had come to get some professional help with Hughes.

Before I started him in day care I was getting some respite, but not enough. I have mentioned that Eric, the mainstay of my support system, took care of his dad at least two days each week for over a year. Also, Hughes was still spending three or four hours twice a week as a volunteer at the county Democratic headquarters. He had been a volunteer for several years with both the state and county offices. The state office had honored him with a Jimmy Carter medallion for his work in mapping the demographics of Democratic voters for the state, and in 1986 he was given the Patriots' Award by the county Democratic Party: "In recognition of a lifelong effort to fulfill America's promise of peace, jobs and justice for all Americans, and in gratitude for the kind of leadership that strives to make our democracy one that truly is of the people, by the people, and for the people." I remember being very anxious when Hughes went up to receive the award because he was then in the "crying phase" of the disease. But he was very brief and made it through all right.

With the onslaught of AD, Hughes went from working with statistics to stuffing envelopes. When he could no longer stuff envelopes, he started sweeping and cleaning the offices. Eventually, of course, he was no longer able to do even that. In a sense, toward the end the county coordinator, Tim Rinne, became Hughes's part-time sitter. Tim had first met Hughes several years before he had AD. As a young VISTA worker fresh out of college, Tim admired Hughes and spent several hours listening to him tell of his life experiences. He has since called Hughes one of his mentors.

After a long talk with Tim, I painfully accepted the fact that Hughes was no longer mentally capable of doing anything at Democratic headquarters. This was a turningpoint for me: I finally decided that I would have to send Hughes to day care at least three days each week.

When I told Eric of my decision, he strongly objected; that was too much like putting his dad in a nursing home. He offered to keep Hughes three days instead of two. At the time, he was single, a university student, and he worked at night. He pleaded with me that he could take the place of the day care. But my mind was made up. Hughes was my responsibility, not his. I also knew that Eric would be graduating soon, and I did not want him building his life around taking care of his dad. (To some extent, he has done so anyway, but that is his choice.)

When I made the decision on day care, I was not sure how I would pay for it, but I was confident there would be a way. At the time Hughes started in December 1988, the cost was $21.68 per day (the national average at that time was about $37); in 1995 it was $30 per day at the center Hughes attends.

Hughes's civil service annuity, which was our retirement income, was sufficient for our frugal way of life so long as we did not get sick but not large enough to accommodate several hundred dollars each month in day-care bills. Throughout our marriage we had always tried to save something from our income, but our savings account remained quite modest. We had put most of our money into our children. They had always been our number one priority, and we had helped each one go to college. Eric, our fourth, would be last to graduate.

I was beginning to see that I was going to have to go back to work in order to have enough each month for Hughes's day-care costs. But I needed to put Hughes in day care *now* and did not think it wise to wait until I got a job. So how would I pay for it? I studied our budget for a long time. Financially, I had to choose between the present and the future, and probably for the first time in my life I chose the present. The future for us was already here.

I decided to drop our high-option health insurance, which cost more than $400 a month, and change to low-option coverage with another company at just under $100. This put enough money back into our budget to start Hughes in day care. Another change I made was to begin taking Hughes to the VA instead of our family physician. I also bought into Medicare for Hughes (at the time he worked for the government, federal employees did not pay into Social Security; thus, he was not automatically eligible for Medicare at age sixty-five).

I tried to cover all the bases for his medical needs, but I knew I was taking a chance with my own health insurance coverage. I was sixty-one at the time, and it would be four more years before I was covered by Medicare, but this was a chance I felt I had to take—a risk I would have to pay for later. In 1992 I had surgery to remove a tumor from my thyroid gland. It was malignant. I had to take treatments, and I have since been declared cancer free. But with only limited health insurance coverage, I had to pay hundreds of dollars out of pocket. (The gamble on my own health almost worked: I had the surgery two months before I turned sixty-five and would have gone on Medicare.) More stressful than learning I had cancer was the immediate ordeal of trying to get correct billing from all of several doctors' offices. There was a time when I was tempted to think that if the cancer didn't kill me, trying to straighten out those bills would. In reality, I tried to take the cancer in stride, relying on my faith to live each day to the fullest.

I told only our children and a few friends about the surgery or the cancer. That was the least stressful way for me. I was in the hospital overnight, and amazingly, Hughes was the only person to notice the scar. He seldom spoke in sentences anymore, but my second night back at home he asked me, "What happened to your neck?"

The first day I took Hughes to day care was the hardest. There is no doubt that he could sense a change taking place that first morning. I had already told him the truth—that he had AD, that I could not take care of him all the time by myself, and that the day-care center was a safe and stimulating place for him to be. Of course, with his short-term memory loss he could not remember what he had just been told. As I drove to the center, I tried to come up with an explanation involving something he liked to do, something that might give him comfort. I decided to tell him he was going to a school where he would be a volunteer helping people. He seemed puzzled and somewhat unsettled, not comforted at all. He wanted to know where I would be and if I was coming back for him. I reassured him over and over again that I would always come back for him.

When we entered the center that first day, the supervisor of the AD unit greeted us warmly and took Hughes by the hand. I felt a lot as I had the first day I took our oldest child, Nena, to school—as if I were losing something or abandoning a loved one. I hated to leave Hughes, but the supervisor assured me he would be just fine. I left in tears, feeling guilty—but only as long as it took me to walk back to my car. As I drove away, I reminded myself that it was insane for me to think I could take care of a demented person twenty-four hours a day, year in and year out, without relief. I also reminded myself that day care would enable me to keep Hughes living at home longer, and after all, that was my objective: to keep him in our home as long as possible. By the time I reached our house, I was at peace about taking Hughes to day care.

The AD day-care center staff keeps a daily journal for each patient, telling about his or her activities. The journal is sent home with the patient. The family then returns it the next time the patient attends, after recording any pertinent information about what has gone on in the interim. The first entry for Hughes, written by the supervisor, read, "12-5-88 Welcome to our program. We really enjoyed Hughes today. Such a kind gentleman. He hummed along to the Christmas music. One of our medical staff brought in his harpsichord. Eric's visit was great. Afterwards, we cut coupons, took a walk and trimmed the tree. Beef roast, potatoes, vegetables, banana, roll and milk for lunch. I'm enclosing a few forms. I need you to help us think of activity ideas. We send a physical info form to doctor."

Each day for the first week when I went to pick Hughes up, I waited for the supervisor to say to me, "Why are you bringing him here? He doesn't belong here. He doesn't act like the other patients with AD." But she never did. My denial was never very far away in those earlier years.

It took Hughes at least a year to adjust to going to day care. At that time he still had some periods of lucidity and often asked as I drove him to the center, "Why are you doing this to me? I wouldn't do this to you." I felt terrible, despite my sensible conversations with myself. I also felt helpless to respond, since dementia cannot reason. All I could do was console myself with the thought deep inside that I was doing what was best for both of us. I would choke back the tears and think, "Now you have to be strong. You have to toughen up." I often meditated on that scripture verse "The Lord is my strength." Almost every day-care morning for that whole year Hughes said adamantly, "I am not going to that place!" But each day I took him anyway. I tried to arrive by nine o'clock, and I picked him up by five in the afternoon (the center was open from seven until five-thirty, Monday through Friday; it is now open on Saturdays as well).

Day care was in fact a blessed relief for both of us. It gave me some days back and the opportunity to make a fresh start—to begin a brand new life. It was exciting and challenging to audition for and be accepted by the speakers' bureau of the local Humanities Council. Since then I have traveled throughout the state, meeting new people and lecturing on African-American history. I have also spoken several times in South Dakota on caregiving, ways for women to become whole, human rights, and Black history.

Day care also gave Hughes a new life. The members of the staff, usually caregivers by choice who have had some training or experience in caring for persons with dementia, were immediately less judgmental and more accepting of Hughes than I was. They were not emotionally involved with him or personally threatened by his deterioration, not having known him before AD. Their ready acceptance and the stimulation of change have helped him retain some minimal skills, despite his continued progression in the disease.

Also, he is freer to move about at the center than at home, since the physical environment is designed and structured specifically for persons with dementia. (Our house is not; though I have made many changes, there are still off-limit areas for his own safety.) The door to the entrance of the center's AD unit can be opened from the inside only with a key. This prevents patients from wandering off. The door can be readily opened from the outside, however, and an exit door to a fenced-in, partially shaded courtyard is always unlocked. There are tables and chairs, a grill, and feeders for the birds and squirrels. The area is also large enough for patients to walk and wander around in and get some exercise.

Patients are served a continental breakfast, a complete meal at noon, and an afternoon snack. Activities include socializing with friends, discussing current events, reminiscing, baking, physical exercises, games, crafts, and bus rides for field trips. The patients also receive frequent visits from children and pets. Each family is asked to provide a biography of the patient with the application, and activities are planned to maximize each individual's strengths and interests. Hughes is evaluated every six months, and I am asked for suggestions about areas I would like the staff to work on with him. Over the years I learned a great deal from the staff about what Hughes could still do, and whatever craft items he became interested in at the center I also bought for our home.

In the earlier years Hughes was mentally capable of participating in several activities. He could put together a puzzle of the United States, cut pictures out of magazines, join in physical exercises, make envelopes, read the newspaper, paint, and so on. Gradually, as he lost these abilities, he began to rearrange the furniture and run the carpet sweeper. Today, he is mostly sedentary both at day care and at home.

Some family members of AD patients have remarked bitterly that they feel it a waste to have to spend their money on day care. I do not share that feeling. Day care has been like an oasis in the desert for Hughes and for me. The costs are now a necessary and integral part of our household budget, as much built in as food and heat and electricity, because AD is now a normal part of our lives. We cannot put our living on hold and wait for some magical time when Hughes no longer has the disease. He has it today, and today is the only time we have in which to live our lives.

When I meet new in-home caregivers who are stressed out and say they cannot afford day care, I suggest to them that anyone who is capable of working twenty-four hours a day around the clock is also capable of finding part-time work to help pay for day care.

The costs per year (depending on the number of days per week) are still less than one-third or one-fourth the costs of nursing home care. Of course, to go to a nursing home, Hughes would have to go on Medicaid, and then the taxpayer would foot the bill. Average nursing home costs for this region range from $24,000 to $36,000 a year.

I believe there is a great need for the owners, managers, and staff of adult day-care centers to inform and educate the public about their existence and what respite service is.[1] A more serious problem, however, is how they define their clientele. A nursing student told me about one center that had a hard time finding clients because, in her words, "They are looking for perfect AD patients."

There are approximately three thousand adult day-care centers in the United States, but not all of them admit AD patients, and only a small number have special AD units. Unless a cure for the disease is found within the next twenty years, the need for AD centers will grow as the baby boomers reach old age. According to a report in the *Journal of American Medicine*, ten thousand adult day-care centers are needed now.[2] Further, with America's communities rapidly aging, AD day-care centers must reevaluate, rethink, and broaden their admission criteria to include patients who are well advanced in the disease. At present there is little or no community support for offering respite service to caregivers of patients in the advanced stages of the disease—probably because some professionals believe that patients in advanced stages belong in a nursing home. (According to an HCFA report dated 4 December 1995, of the 1,538,462 residents in nursing facilities and skilled nursing facilities in the United States, 602,946 were classified under "senile dementia or chronic, organic brain syndrome."[3]) But this is a decision that only a family can make, and the informal caregivers apparently disagree with the professionals, since 70 to 80 percent of AD patients are still cared for in their homes. If adult day-care centers can care for helpless young adults, why not helpless old adults?

I know a woman named Helen, in her early sixties, who takes care of her ninety-six-year-old mother, Bessie, who has AD. Three years ago, Bessie was dismissed from the day-care center that she had attended for several years on the grounds that she was too fragile to continue. Yet although Bessie is very slow now, she is still able to walk, and since she was dismissed from the center, Helen has taken her on two plane trips to family reunions in California. This year, she packed up and took her mother first to Florida and then to California for the winter. Helen said she had worked hard all her life and had always wanted to take her mother to a warm climate. She did not feel that her mother's AD, even in the advanced stage, was a reason not to carry out her plans. She and Bessie were renting a furnished condominium in a retirement community; Helen took her mother walking every day and said that Bessie could now walk as much as two blocks.

PAID SITTERS IN THE HOME

I have used paid sitters in a variety of ways. For instance there were times when Hughes was deep in the confusion of the second stage of AD, and I was so exhausted that I felt I had to have immediate relief in order to keep going. On those occasions, a sitter came in for a few mornings to get Hughes ready for day care and to drop him off at the center, allowing me to stay in bed; sometimes I slept all day. At other times, when I felt I had to have a break from the stress of struggling with Hughes every night just to get him undressed and bathed and into bed, a sitter came in for two or three evenings and took over those chores while I went upstairs out of hearing range and read or sewed. In those desperate times, just knowing all day that I would not have to face the usual stress of the evening gave me comfort and relief.

If I had made costs my first consideration, I would never have hired a sitter at all, and I have often had to use savings to pay for such relief. But that is what savings are for—emergencies; and when the primary caregiver is stressed out, it is an emergency. I know an eighty-year-old caregiver who coped by having a sitter come in the mornings and get his wife ready for day care, then return in the evening to give the patient her supper and put her to bed. The husband told me this eliminated his stress.

Still, because of the cost, I try not to hire a sitter unless it is absolutely necessary. Sitters are usually paid by the hour at the rate of $5.00 to $8.00. Colleges usually have an employment officer who could assist community members to find students who want part-time employment (see the section on student interns, below). There are also agencies, usually listed in the local telephone book, that provide paraprofessional help; they may charge $10 to $15 per hour, sometimes more. Paraprofessionals who are available on holidays such as Christmas and Thanksgiving are paid time and a half.

I do recommend hiring a sitter to be on hand for any big family gathering when people have not seen each other for a long time. If the patient needs to be toileted or put to bed, family members do not have to leave the festivities unless they choose to do so. The sitter is there to take care of the patient's needs. At Eric and Sherry's wedding and reception, for example, having a sitter who was specifically in charge of Hughes took the pressure off the rest of us—especially Eric on his special day.

Occasionally, if I must be away, I have to pay someone to come in at night and stay with Hughes. It is important, however, that everyone who makes demands on the caregiver's time outside the home be sensitive to the caregiver's need to provide for the patient in her or his absence. I have had million-dollar businesses and profitmaking institutions ask me to speak on caregiving—often at night and in locations that required driving long distances—free of charge; this is highly inconsiderate, for when the patient needs twenty-four-hour care, the caregiver has to pay someone to take his or her place. (Ask the IRS about employment taxes.)

I have found it wise to have at least three different sitters on call. Once when I was scheduled to talk at a local church and my sitter did not show up, there was no time to call another and I had to take Hughes with me. I explained my circumstances to the chairperson, and she asked Brenda, a member of the congregation who was a nurse, to look after Hughes. He sat quietly for about the first fifteen minutes, but then he got up and walked to the pulpit. Fortunately, Brenda was able to lead him outside, and when I finished speaking, I found them walking peacefully back and forth around the church.

A SHORT STAY WITH A PROFESSIONAL CAREGIVER OR
IN A NURSING HOME

Some caregivers, in order to take a vacation or in the case of other family illness, pay to have the AD patient cared for in a professional's home. Costs for this service can vary from $500 for one week to $1,200 for one month. I have not yet used such a service, but I know caregivers who have found it satisfactory. Some nursing homes too will accept short-term patients, usually for a minimum of one week; count on paying at least $100 a day.

It should be noted, though, that even a brief stay in a totally foreign environment, with a stranger or among unfamiliar staff and residents, can be catastrophic for some AD patients. For one who normally attends a center during the day, however, the trauma of change might be lessened by planning for his or her transportation each day to the familiar faces and environment of the day care center. This arrangement provides some stability and continuity in routine, staff, and environment for the patient in the absence of the family.

DONATED SERVICES

Not all caregivers have enough income or savings to pay for fee-based respite services. Where can they look for help?

A STUDENT INTERN IN THE HOME

The first sitter I found for Hughes was a young man who was majoring in sociology at a nearby university. Our friend Nan was on the faculty there, and she inquired of a colleague in the sociology department whether such an internship might be possible. He asked his students if anyone was interested, and Rob volunteered. He came once a week for at least two hours during one semester. In addition to sitting and talking with Hughes, he learned how to assist with his bath and get him ready for bed. He was Hughes's primary sitter for the next two years, until he graduated.

The second person to serve an internship with Hughes was Brian, a college senior majoring in communications. His career goal is to work as a consultant with doctors to help them better understand how to communicate with all kinds of persons who might become their patients.

Since a beginning caregiver is often too tired and traumatized to know where to begin looking for suitable help, it would be useful for local support groups or social services departments in areas where there are colleges and universities to develop and maintain a current list of possible interns (as well as paid student caregivers). In addition to the sociology department, contacts could be made with nursing, gerontology, psychology, human services, and other departments. In the absence of a college, high school students who want to go into nursing and medicine are possibilities. Support groups and social workers could consult with high school counselors in developing a list of prospective interns (or paid sitters).

A FRIEND OR FAMILY MEMBER IN THE HOME

In the early days, both before and after I started Hughes in day care, Eric was my primary sitter; he also came several mornings and evenings and helped with his dad. One of my most treasured Mother's Days came in 1989 when Eric told me that my present was the entire day off from Hughes's care. I did exactly what I wanted to do that one day. First, I dressed up, then I spent the day in the public library. I was able to finish writing the script for my first video documentary on Hughes and AD, which aired on public access television.

I looked to Eric for relief, but I also learned to ask for and use the help of people outside our family. Eventually, I began putting Hughes in day care five days a week, but before that our friend Rita would drop by, often unexpectedly, and announce that I could take off. What bliss! She usually came on Sunday afternoons after I had been with Hughes all weekend. Respite service is the most valuable gift one can give the caregiver.

In 1990, 1993, and 1995, Cedric came for a week and took care of his dad so that I could have a real vacation. In 1990, I did not have the strength or energy to leave town, so I moved into a local motel for the week. All I wanted to do was sleep and rest and have some time to visit with Cedric; we talked each day and often met for lunch. But in 1993 I went to Sewickley, Pennsylvania, to visit our daughter Shela and our son-in-law Jim and our four grandchildren: Orpheus, Zenith, Zoë, and Orchid. This was the first time I had seen Orchid, who was then two years old. In 1995 I used my time off to attend the Alzheimer's Association's annual Public Policy Forum in Washington DC.

Hughes did not know Cedric during these weeks. That was difficult for our son to take in 1990; when he first arrived and saw that his dad no longer recognized him, he cried. But one night as Cedric was tucking him into bed, Hughes looked at him and said, "Thank you. You are doing a good job."

When Cedric is here, I insist that Hughes still attend day care. This gives him continuity and stability, and it allows Cedric to spend most of his days making necessary home repairs.

In November 1993, Shela came and took care of her dad over Thanksgiving weekend. Of course, he did not know her either. But I now understand better how to prepare our family and friends for a visit with Hughes. I usually say to visitors before they come, "Hughes looks a lot like he always did in outer appearance. His eyes are bright and he often smiles. It is easy to think when we look at him, "Now, he could remember if he really tried." But he cannot remember because the connectors in his brain are broken. If you are not accepting him, though, he will know it on the inside, and this will cause him great anxiety, great unrest, and great pain. That is why it is essential to accept him as he is while you are here. He is still sweet, kind, and gentle. He is still a charmer, and in an atmosphere of acceptance, he will give you his love."

FAMILY MEMBERS WHO SHARE IN CAREGIVING

Some families may find it best for members to take turns caring for their loved one in their homes. Hughes's sisters, for example, alternated in caring for their mother for several years. Unfortunately, they did not have the benefit of adult day-care centers.

I know of other families, however, where only one of several grown children will take the AD parent into his or her home to prevent institutionalization. In one case in particular, when the caregiver, who is a schoolteacher, wants a much-needed respite, rarely will any of her several siblings take their mother in, or at best they do so grudgingly. Their attitude is that the mother belongs in a nursing home, and therefore they feel no responsibility for her care. Granted, there are many reasons why not everyone is able to be a caregiver, but in such a case, siblings could voluntarily pay for a sitter once a year while the primary caregiver takes time off.

One daughter, who has taken care of her eighty-seven-year-old mother for the past six years, said of her siblings: "I have five brothers and sisters, and when I first brought mother to be with me, I spent a lot of time and energy trying to get them involved in the caregiving. It became so draining on me that I just decided I would accept whatever help they chose to give and not allow myself to become bitter or have it affect the way I treated mother. I have found that it is possible to take care of my mother and still work full time. I do this in free will and with lots of love. I feel fortunate to still have mother with us. I call it a precious duty."

AN OUTING WITH A FRIEND OR FAMILY MEMBER

In the early days, our good friends Cynthia and Elden took Hughes on Sunday outings. They went to flower shows and for long drives. Les, our friend of many years, took Hughes to a monthly dinner meeting until he became too confused to be out at night. Eric often dropped by unexpectedly and took Hughes along for the ride while he ran errands. I welcomed and appreciated any consideration of this sort.

THE STATE DEPARTMENT OF SOCIAL SERVICES

One federal program in cooperation with the states is called "Medicaid Home and Community-Based Services Waivers for the Elderly." Under this program, forty-four states are providing a range of services to persons who might otherwise be relegated to institutional care. According to *Eldercare in the Home and Community*, December 1992, "The services may include, but are not limited to, case management, homemaker services, personal care, day care, habilitation services, and respite services. Services offered through the Medicaid waivers program may be limited to a specific population group, such as the elderly, or to persons living in a particular geographic area of the state. States providing home and community-based services under a waiver must meet certain cost-effectiveness standards set by HCFA."[4]

Before the Medicaid Waivers bill was passed, a family's income had to be at poverty or near-poverty level before the disabled aged could qualify for such services; despite his disability, Hughes's income would have made him ineligible. Now, however, it gives me some comfort and relief to know that I can apply for these services if I ever need to.

PART FOUR
Hopes
and
Rewards

TEN

The Future for Alzheimer's Patients and Caregivers

Hughes is one of four members of his family to have an irreversible dementia. In addition to his mother, his younger brother Charlie has AD, and his oldest sibling, Emily, died from AD while I was writing this book. As a mother and grandmother, I have felt helpless when our children and grandchildren have wondered aloud if they too will get this disease. As a caregiver and as an aging American, I have felt the need to find answers as to what the future may hold for my children and other families of AD patients.

It has been estimated that by the year 2030, 22 percent of the population will be sixty-five and older, and "the prevalence of severe dementia rises steeply with age."[1] Further, the number of persons eighty-five and older is projected to be nearly seven times larger by 2050 than it was in 1980, and at present persons over the age of eighty-five account for 47 percent of people with AD. By the year 2050 "an estimated 14 million Americans will have AD unless medical research finds a way to prevent or slow the progress of the disease," according to the Chicago-based Alzheimer's Association.[2] This projection more than triples today's approximate number of four million persons with the disease.

Moreover, AD is the third costliest disease in the nation, exceeded only by heart disease and cancer. Families and patients pay most of the expenses. For each person with AD, the cost of home care nationwide averaged about $18,000 in 1992, and nursing home care approximately $50,000. Alzheimer's cost the nation $67.3 billion in 1991, including medical expenses, round-the-clock care, and lost productivity.[3] Projected total costs for the future care of persons with AD are estimated to reach into the trillions of dollars.

But despite these dire predictions, the future looks much brighter for members of my children's generation, the baby boomers, who might get AD. In fact, since some patients live as long as twenty years with the disease, Hughes may yet live to receive some benefit from scientific research. Changes (some faster than others) are occurring in several areas that could directly affect the lives and the quality of life of persons who have the disease. I can now tell my children about progress in four broad areas: medical and scientific research, the nursing home industry, technology, and public policy.

MEDICAL AND SCIENTIFIC RESEARCH

The most dramatic changes are taking place in medical and scientific research, since it is through scientific discoveries that the disease may be stopped from spreading to other members of our family. The Alzheimer's Association, which has 212 local chapters, has led the way as the largest funder outside the federal government of Alzheimer's research. The association lists five goals for the treatment of AD: "managing or preventing behavioral symptoms, improving cognitive symptoms, slowing or stopping the progression of the disease, delaying the onset of symptoms, and preventing the disease altogether."[4]

According to Dr. Eric Pfeiffer, director of the National Eldercare Institute on Long Term Care and Alzheimer's Disease at the Suncoast Gerontology Center, University of South Florida, "Researchers are working furiously on drugs to slow AD." Forty different drugs either to slow down or to reverse the disease are being tested.[5]

Already, some persons have been helped by taking Cognex, the brand name for the drug tactrine, which was approved for general distribution in October 1993 by the U.S. Food and Drug Administration. As a caregiver, I know that the smallest improvement in an AD patient is significant to the family. For example, it would be of unimaginable help to me if Hughes could perform any one of the basic ADLs such as putting on his shirt or pants or socks or shoes. (He does occasionally *remove* his socks and shoes, usually at inappropriate times.) Cognex has improved some patient's memory and "appears to stop the progression of the disease." Unfortunately, only 20 to 30 percent of AD patients made any improvement after taking Cognex.[6] Moreover, it was tested only on persons with mild to moderate symptoms, and it also has some possible side effects including liver damage, but that can be monitored by testing the patient's blood on a regular basis to measure liver enzymes. Dr. Pfeiffer states that a drug is now being tested that is similar to Cognex but does not have the side effects.

Several other drugs are now in clinical trials: physostigmine, to jump the gap in nerve transmissions; deprenyl, to slow the progression of the disease. Estrogen, a hormone, and indomethacin, an antiinflammatory drug, "have been shown in recent small studies to delay the onset of the disease and reduce its effects."[7] Also, nerve growth factor (NGF), a chemical in the body, is "considered to have great theoretical potential for treating AD."[8] It is exciting to contemplate that the brain might be able to repair its damaged nerve cells.

In addition to drug research, the discovery of a genetic link, announced in 1992 and 1993, was considered a major breakthrough in AD scientific research. Dr. Allen D. Roses, a neurobiologist at Duke University in Durham, North Carolina, led the team of scientists who made this discovery. The gene involved is called apolipoprotein E e4 (ApoE e4), and the findings have been confirmed by several other researchers. Dr. Roses explains, "Having this particular form of the gene doesn't mean that you're going to get AD; not having it doesn't mean that you won't get AD. From what we have seen so far, it seems that this gene is more than twice as common in Alzheimer patients as it is in the general population, which suggests that a person who has it has a greater likelihood of developing AD, whether or not anyone else in the family has had the disease."[9]

It should be noted that since not all persons with AD have this gene, other factors must be involved in developing the disease. Scientists do not know yet exactly what they are—some point to head trauma and aging itself as risk factors—but are hoping that "a greater understanding of the ApoE gene can help them identify controllable risk factors for AD." Dr. Roses speculates that "in the future, identifying the type of ApoE gene a person has may be as routine as measuring blood cholesterol to assess risk for heart disease." He states, "I am absolutely convinced that within ten years we will have a pill that prevents AD." Dr. Roses is now working with British scientists from the pharmaceutical company Glaxo Holdings PLC to try to develop a drug for Alzheimer's based on his discoveries. In addition, by September 1995 a total of three genes showing a possible family link had been identified.

The first "test" for determining genetic susceptibility to AD has been marketed by the Genica Pharmaceuticals Corporation of Worcester, Massachusetts. This is a risk factor assessment called the ApoE GenoType Report, said to have a "greater than 99 percent accuracy." According to Genica, it "does not identify anyone as having, or not having, AD. In fact, the ApoE GenoType Report is not a "test." Rather, Genica is offering a genotyping service that identifies the likelihood that a particular patient's symptoms of idiopathic dementia are caused by AD."[10] Dr. Pfeiffer, at the Suncoast Gerontology Center, recommends that any such testing be done only through an AD research center, since a private physician may not be able to interpret the results accurately.

At the National Institute of Neurological Disorders and Stroke, biophysicist Daniel Alkon is conducting tests to determine whether AD can be diagnosed through a simple skin test, or if "a skin test might one day be used to predict whether or not a person will develop Alzheimer's."[11] I am not sure, however, that I would want to be tested for potential AD until there is a cure).

Researchers are also trying to find a "biological marker" for AD: that is, "some component of a person's body, such as a protein or other substance, that can be measured to determine whether a person has a particular disease." Such a marker would greatly simplify the diagnosis of AD. Several international research groups are collaborating on how to improve and standardize the methods being used to diagnose the disease and "to develop a detailed database of the characteristics of patients with AD."[12]

THE NURSING HOME INDUSTRY

There is probably nothing more painful for a caregiver than the decision to put a loved one in a nursing home. Yet the necessity of nursing home placement can become a reality for any of us. Despite wealth, class, race, education, or station in life, if we live long enough, we are all vulnerable to aging and disease. After Hughes was diagnosed with AD, I confronted the possibility not just for him but also for myself, and I took out a nursing home insurance policy.

When I first registered Hughes in several nursing homes, I knew nothing about models of care or how they differ one from the other. Mainly, all I knew was that some homes were odiferous and some were not. I felt strongly that I needed to know more in order to make an intelligent and wise decision in the future. I have since learned that most nursing homes are structured on the medical model, the "sick" model, but that the nursing home industry all over the world is slowly moving toward a social model. This change can be very beneficial for many AD patients.

A nursing home on the medical model, usually patterned after the design and plan of a hospital, is set up to treat and (if possible) cure people who are physically ill.[13] It is staffed by health professionals who are trained to treat whatever disease or infirmity each patient has. But with today's improved medical technology, the elderly are living not only longer but healthier lives. We also know now that despite physical changes as we grow older, disease and illness are not synonymous with aging.[14] And although AD is a disease primarily of the aged, not only is there very little medical treatment available, but "many in the early and middle stages of the disease are physically active and not in need of extensive medical care."[15] (Hughes is the perfect example. In fact at his six-month checkup this year, his doctor commented that there had been no change in his physical health in the several years he has been Hughes's physician.) Yet in the medical model it is not uncommon for the staff to give drugs to physically active AD patients for the specific purpose of immobilizing them.[16] The design of the facility and the training and understanding of the staff are seldom adequate to handle the social behavior of the person with AD.[17]

By contrast, the outstanding characteristic of the social model is that it is interdisciplinary and is designed and planned around all of each patient's needs and strengths: social, psychological, physical, and spiritual.[18] In the social model the person with a dementia is accepted as a unique individual with a life story, rather than as a problem patient. Medical treatment is not the focal point but one of many services provided to the residents. All the components in the social model are used therapeutically for the patient, including the design of the physical structure, the programs and activities, and the interactions of each staff member with each patient. Moyra J. D. Jones of Burnaby, British Columbia, speaks of one example, called Gentlecare, as "a prosthetic system of care designed to support the person with dementia rather than challenge them."[19]

Within facilities structured on the social model, however, there is a wide range of modalities. For example, some special-care units plan programs and outside activities for the residents, whereas Gentlecare, focuses principally on promoting the residents' self-care: eating, dressing, grooming, bathing, and toileting. Planned programs and field trips are deemed to be too stressful and challenging.

A unique example of the social model is the Eden Alternative at Chase Memorial Nursing Home in New Berlin, New York, where the lobby has an aviary. According to Medical Director William Thomas, M.D., the home has eighty residents, ninety birds, two dogs, four cats, and hundreds of growing plants. Outside there are two rabbits and a flock of laying hens complete with a rooster. (The campus also has a day-care center, an after-school program, and a summer camp for children of the community.) In place of a lawn, there are wildflower meadows and vegetable and flower gardens; many of the residents work along with the gardener to help plant, cultivate, and harvest the vegetables. The "core concept" of Eden Alternative, according to Dr. Thomas, is that nursing homes should be "habitats for human beings rather than institutions for the frail and elderly. . . . The Eden Alternative seeks to eliminate the three plagues of long term care institutions—loneliness, helplessness and boredom. We want to show others how companion animals, the opportunity to care for other living things and the variety and spontaneity that mark an enlivened environment can succeed where pills and therapies fail."[20] Other nursing homes on the social model may occasionally have "pet therapy," "intergenerational programming," and "horticulture therapy," but these are everyday occurrences at Chase Memorial.

Whatever the differences within the social model, certain general features or characteristics clearly distinguish it from the medical model.

PHILOSOPHY OF CARE

Residents live in small family-style groups with persons of similar cognitive abilities. Each resident is treated as an individual, and his or her life history is known by all staff. In addition, each staff member has the responsibility of knowing and following each resident's comprehensive care plan. (According to OSCAR Report 18, the second highest violation in the nation's nursing homes was not developing a comprehensive care plan for each resident.) Mary Buzzell, director of community relations, Victorian Order of Nurses, Hamilton-Wentworth, Ontario, Canada, states that it is more important to know the person's history than to know the diagnosis.[21]

The language and the attitude toward patients change in the social model. In fact, they are called "residents" rather than "patients," and the staff is there to give support, not to "manage" or "control" them. Director Jones states that Gentlecare staff try not to change the behavior of the residents but to "help them live with the consequences of the illness."

Susan Gilster, director of the Alois Alzheimer Center in Cincinnati, Ohio, thinks it is important to create an environment and an atmosphere that avoid crisis: "If you employ an obsessive, compulsive professional that has to run around and create crisis, I would suggest, having learned the hard way, that you get rid of that person as fast as you can."[22] Chari Weber, director of the Nason Center in Breckenridge Village, Cleveland, Ohio, advocates "setting up models that avoid placing the staff in a position of feeling they have to control patients or that residents [are] inept or incapable." She speaks of turning problems into programs.[23] Nurse Buzzell recommends using the term "lifecare" in place of "long-term care," which "connotes for many people problems and deficits." She hopes that thinking of "lifecare" will put the focus on the person and the family.

The daily schedule is more flexible in the social model, in order to accommodate the desires of the residents. According to gerontologist Dorothy

Coons, people with AD "are strongly resistive to the rigid schedules" of traditional nursing homes.[24] One feature of the Gentlecare model is called "Flexible Care Routine": residents get up when they wake up, eat when they wish, go to bed and carry out their daily activities on their own personal schedule. According to Moyra Jones, under such a routine there is less catastrophe behavior, incontinence is reduced, family comfort is enhanced, staff morale is better, and costs go down.

Another major difference from the medical model is that the social model discourages the use of chemicals and restraints as means of controlling the patients. In some facilities they are eliminated altogether.

Care is provided on a continuum in this model. This means that most facilities provide some or all of the services needed by persons with dementia, from the onset of the disease to the end. Services begin with AD adult day care. Some facilities also offer short-stay respite service so that families can take a vacation from caregiving; patients spend the night in the short-stay wing of the facility, but during the day they can attend the adult day-care center they are already used to, with its familiar staff and familiar environment. When the family feels it can no longer care for the person in the home, the patient is placed in long-term care in specialized AD units or cottages. In the cottage model, residents move to the appropriate cottage as they progress in the disease; in some facilities, members of the staff move with the residents. When patients are no longer ambulatory, they are placed in the skilled nursing unit of the facility.

PHYSICAL STRUCTURES

In the social model, residents live in structures designed specifically to accommodate and support persons with dementia. The intent is to create the atmosphere of a home in every way possible. Some older nursing homes that are in transition from the medical model to the social model are designating a "special care unit" (SCU) in one part of the existing structure. Unfortunately, says Dorothy Coons, "in many cases the units can make no claims to being special except that they are segregating persons who are bothersome to other residents and staff. Some facilities merely relabel units that have been segregated in the past." Ivy Winchester, administrator of Williamsburg Villas, Knoxville, Tennessee, cautions, "It's not going to be enough anymore to lock a wing in a nursing home and place an Alzheimer's unit sign outside of it and call yourself a specialty unit."[25]

Since 1986, Rhode Island has had a statewide demonstration project to assist public and private long-term care facilities in developing special-care units. E. Paul Larrat, assistant professor at the University of Rhode Island College of Pharmacy, points out that "the effectiveness of SCU's in improving the quality of life . . . for residents is still widely debated . . . but several research studies . . . have noted improvements in cognition and functional ability among residents of special care units."[26]

Some institutions successfully refurbish old buildings. A former elementary school was renovated for the Alois Alzheimer Center in Cincinnati. According to its director, the center is designed to "maximize the residents' capabilities and minimize the disabilities," allowing them to maintain functional levels for long periods of time.

Other entrepreneurs build self-contained cottages where ten to sixteen residents live with the staff. These group homes are designed like a private home with several bedrooms, private or semiprivate, and patients are expected and encouraged to personalize their rooms. Some bring familiar furniture from home and hang pictures on the walls. Many cottages include a living room with a fireplace. Each cottage also has several activity rooms to accommodate various levels of activities simultaneously. Both the cottages and the special-care units are designed for maximum natural sunlight.

Design principles include rounded windows—a shape unlike that of windows in most houses and public buildings—to cue residents that they are in a different place but not in a hospital; Dutch doors; table edges clearly marked; contrasting colors between chairs and floors, and between light switches and walls. Making toilet entrances more visible and accessible is also an improved characteristic in the social model. Some centers use privacy curtains instead of doors. The curtains can be closed when the toilet is in use but are otherwise pulled back and kept open so that residents can see the toilet.

Security is important for the AD patient, and in the social model it is built into the design in many ways, including clear differences between entrances and exits that are accessible to residents and those that are not. Wandering paths with handrails are often circular, bringing walkers back to their starting point. In some centers the wandering paths have an area for snacks along the way. The paths may be interior, following the perimeter of the structure, or may extend to a secured wandering track and garden outside. In one center in Sydney, Australia, all rooms open out to the garden area. This is in sharp contrast to the old medical model where residents given to wandering were strapped in chairs.[27] Gilster states that when persons are "content, and they are happy and they feel accomplished, and they feel good about who they are, then they do not have the need to escape. If it looks like I can go anytime I want to, there is not a sense of confinement." Jones confirms that many of the residents in Gentlecare are "walking around until they die." She believes there "can be a different end if we give them different care."[28]

STAFFING AND TRAINING

The person in charge in the social model is often an activity coordinator rather than a nurse, and the hub of activity is the activity room or living area. A nurse is always on duty, of course, but the nursing station is usually a room out of sight of the central activity area.

Training and education of staff, family, and community members are built into the facility's programming. At the Alois Alzheimer Center, educational programs for staff on all three shifts have been held once a week for more than six years. At Gentlecare, all persons who come in contact with the residents, including the cook and the housekeeper, receive intensive training about dementia and are expected to be able to interact therapeutically with all the residents. At Wesley Gardens in Sydney, Australia, there are "no designated roles for staff" but instead a "blending of staff."[29]

Some new facilities using the social model have a policy of not hiring nurses who have worked in a medical model nursing home in the previous two years. According to Jacqueline M. Stolley, a certified gerontological nurse, a nurse assigned to dementia patients but untrained in the symptoms of the disease, whether in a hospital or a nursing facility, can have catastrophic consequences for the patients.[30]

FAMILY INVOLVEMENT

There is more family and community involvement in the social model. In some nursing homes on the medical model, family members are asked not to visit a loved one with AD for the first few weeks after he or she is admitted. In the social model, family and community members are encouraged to become volunteers, and some facilities feel a responsibility to provide information and training to the community about the disease. For example, Wesley Gardens has an ongoing training program for staff, and this training is offered free of charge to AD organizations as well.

TECHNOLOGY

In addition to nursing home changes and medical advances, new technology is improving the lives of the cognitively impaired through assistive

devices and environmental interventions that can postpone institutionalization and also relieve the burden of caregivers. At present there are at
least 25,000 assistive devices available to all types of consumers who need
some form of assistance, according to Dianne Hurren of the Rehabilitation
Engineering Research Center on Aging at the University of Buffalo in New
York.[31] Among the devices now in use to aid persons in various stages of
dementia are a memory dial phone, an intercom system, a bath lift and a
bed lift, a stair glide, and a plastic lever-style door handle.

In fact, in an assessment study of cognitively impaired persons and their
caregivers, the center in Buffalo discovered that "almost every device people listed that they'd like to see developed is already available in the mar-
ketplace, but the caregivers don't know of [their] availability, or where to
purchase them, or [whether] they cannot afford them." As a result of the
study, the center developed "Project Link," which assists consumers in identifying and locating assistive devices they may need. ("Project Link" can be
reached at 1-800-628-2281.) Further, an interdisciplinary team at the center is researching the use of high-tech and low-tech devices. High-tech products include an electronic alerting device, a computerized medication system, and a voice-activated phone. Low-tech products include lists and signs
on doors to jog memory, like those I used with Hughes in the earlier stages
of the disease. Hurren states that the center is working on a "universal design" for products that the general population could also use, thus cutting
down on costs and reducing the stigma attached to assistive devices.

The consumer assessment study revealed that one physical device caregivers need is something to assist the AD person in getting in and out of
the car. I recognize this real need almost every time I try to get Hughes into
the car; in fact, there are days when I prefer walking the five miles to and
from the day-care center rather than trying to do so. Some progress has
been made; medical supply stores have "transfer boards" for sliding patients
from one chair or seat to another, and disks for shifting their feet.

PUBLIC POLICY

Public policy has slowly moved toward giving greater support to caregivers who provide twenty-four-hour care at home, as well as those who
oversee the care of patients in nursing homes.

To date, none of Hughes's respite care services are covered under Medicare or our Blue Cross and Blue Shield federal employee program. In fact,
by 1993 our out-of-pocket health care expenses—including respite service,

all health insurance premiums, dentist and doctor bills not covered by our health insurance, medications, and medical supplies—totaled over one-half of his federal annuity. If I were to divide between us what we have left, our income would put us at the poverty level.

Most countries have historically resisted including nonmedical long-term care in their health programs, or giving any financial support to families that provide long-term care in the home. Today, however, with people living longer throughout the developed countries and health care costs in crisis, policymakers in western Europe and North America are beginning to acknowledge the contribution of in-home caregivers and considering the implications of a drastic rise in health care costs without them. As Lynn B. Gerald, research associate in the Department of Sociology and Anthropology at the University of South Alabama, points out, "Supporting caregivers in their difficult task can prevent premature or unnecessary institutionalization of the elderly and cut the rising costs of medical care to the institutionalized elderly."[32] Forty-four states provided services under the Medicaid Home and Community-Based Services Waivers in 1992.[33]

In 1993 the 103d Congress passed the Family and Medical Leave Act (PL 103-3), which requires employers with fifty or more workers to allow an employee up to twelve weeks of unpaid, job-protected leave to care for a newborn or adopted child, a sick child, spouse, or parent, or because of the employee's own serious health condition.[34] Canada, Sweden, the Netherlands, and the United Kingdom also provide some form of support for caregivers. Sweden probably has "the most comprehensive family caregiving support program in the world."[35] Its features include a federal leave policy, salaries for full-time family caregivers, and job training for caregivers when their caregiving tasks end.

Research shows low utilization of available services in the United States, however.[36] I understand that; like me, many caregivers prefer to remain as independent and self-sufficient as possible. Further, when respite services are provided through the Medicaid Waivers program, caregivers do not always have control over who comes into their home to take care of their loved one; a patient might even have a different health care worker each time. This causes stress for both patient and caregiver. But despite the problems and difficulties, caregivers do need a safety net. Someday I may be happy to use the services of the waivers program—if they have not been cut.

In the workplace, some employers are gradually providing more support for their employees who are also caregivers. For example, in 1990 the Stride Rite Corporation opened an intergenerational day-care center at its headquarters in Cambridge, Massachusetts. The center is designed to provide day care to both children and elders in the same facility and accepts persons with early onset AD. Some companies are also offering on-site support group meetings or personal counseling, or contracting with private firms to help employees manage care for relatives in distant cities.

Over the years since Hughes developed AD, my greatest needs have been information, counseling, training, and respite service—in that order. Now and in the future, physicians and diagnostic clinics should provide patients' families with a comprehensive informational packet on the disease at the time of diagnosis. And until a cure is found, there should be ongoing weekly training programs for caregivers for every stage of the disease, organized and run by a private or public entity. Just as a doctor refers a cancer patient to an oncologist, ideally the doctor who diagnoses AD would recommend or make an appointment for the family with a counselor at a formal training center where they can receive information, help, understanding, and support. "Upon diagnosis of Alzheimer's disease . . . it would be humane and medically appropriate for the attending physician to prescribe: Rehabilitation Care for the dementia patient and Retreat for their family caregiver," according to Joy Glenner, executive director of the George G. Glenner Alzheimer's Family Centers in San Diego, and Lorie Van Tilburg, executive director of the Southern Caregiver Resource Center, San Diego.[37]

It should be noted that local Alzheimer's Association chapters do provide periodic workshops and training sessions for caregivers, along with weekly, biweekly, or monthly support group meetings. Certain segments of the caregiver population, however, tend not to join traditional support groups, including some males and some African Americans and other ethnic minorities.[38] In addition, the ongoing needs of caregivers are too constant and often too desperate to rely on periodic informal training. When Hughes was in the beginning stage, my greatest help came from our weekly visits to Chris Milne, the VA psychologist, but that kind of help is not available to everyone. Since "Alzheimer's disease will be the public health crisis of the 21st century," according to the Alzheimer's Association,[39] there should be a national social policy encouraging and supporting, through matching federal grants, the opening of formalized caregiver training centers.

Doctors can help, as the Council on Scientific Affairs of the American Medical Association stated in a 1991 report: "Primary care physicians need a strong and effective model to guide their relationships with family caregivers. . . . Caregivers provide a significant proportion of the home care needed by the rapidly growing number of frail elderly living in the community. Caregiving exacts a physical, psychological, social, and emotional toll that no intervention strategies have proven powerful enough to offset. An effective relationship model would acknowledge the key linkage role of the primary care physician, recognize that caregivers and patients form interdependent units, and affirm a care partnership between the physician and caregiver. In this model, the physician . . . provides training to caregivers, particularly in managing difficult behavior.[40]

There are some training manuals for AD caregivers; those available on microfiche include "Alzheimer's Disease Family Support Groups, An Education and Training Manual" (U.S. Department of Health and Human Services, December 1986); "Alzheimer's Disease In-Home Respite Care Training Curriculum Guide," Lillian Middleton, M.S.W., Editor and Project Director (U.S. Department of Health and Human Services, 1987, developed by the University of South Florida Suncoast Gerontology Center, Tampa, Florida); and "Alzheimer's Disease: Pieces of the Puzzle, a Training Program for Direct Service Staff and Family Caregivers" (U.S. Department of Health and Human Services, 1990, developed by the Arizona Long Term Care Gerontology Center at the Arizona Health Sciences Center, University of Arizona). The best way to locate these is to inquire at the nearest university library or the local public library. In addition, many local AD associations offer caregiver training manuals, and I have outlined a training model (see the appendix) based on my individual needs over the years.

Hubert Humphrey, the late senator and vice-president, once said, "The measure of a society is how it treats those in the dawn of life, the children; the twilight of life, the aged; the shadow of life, the sick and the needy."[41] The verdict is still out on America as we grapple with how to fix the health care system and its escalating costs. These are ongoing issues that are debated in the Congress over and over again. Each generation in turn must face health care concerns. I do not believe that my generation—the generation that changed the world through the 1960s civil rights movement—will let Medicare and Medicaid wither on the vine without a fight. We were mere babes in the 1960s. Today we are experienced warriors.

Whatever happens in the health care system, however—and despite advances in research, technology, and nursing home procedures—AD patients are still judged primarily by the standards of cognitive ability and economic productivity, not for their humanity and inner spirit. There is still no national social policy on AD, and ultimately, caregivers who make the decision to keep their loved ones at home must be prepared to face the costs and the consequences on their own.

Yet as a civilized society and the richest nation in the world, we have a responsibility to expand our vision of health care to include all the helpless among us. We are interdependent as individuals, as a nation, and as a world. A nation that abandons its most vulnerable is a nation without a soul. All we need is the vision and the will.

ELEVEN
The New Life of the Caregiver and Its Rewards

The years since 1984 have been a long, hard, arduous journey. There have been more mountains to climb than I could have imagined in our two lifetimes. My sweet prince, the father of my children, has returned in giant form to his childhood. The love of my life as I once knew him is lost to me forever. Life is also merciful, and my years as a caregiver have never been without their rewards. Yet making the break from Hughes physically and emotionally while he was (and still is) a strong, vibrant human being has taken lots of time, constant effort, and a steely determination.

It has been especially difficult because I was part of a generation that grew up on romance. It was a time when a woman was nothing without a man. We were in love with love. We read the true love story magazines. We sang the lyrics "I only live for your love and your kiss," and "Because of you, my life is now worthwhile." Only in retrospect can we see that we were living in a fantasyland, looking for an idyllic state that never existed anywhere in the world except in our romantic daydreams.

In some ways, our courtship and marriage had been like the love songs and the storybook romance, or so I thought—until we got to this part. We had been constant companions, friends, and lovers for two-thirds of my life. Now that was over. On the one hand Hughes was still here with me, but on the other hand he was not. Some people have referred to AD spouse caregivers as widows and widowers without the death, and one writer has stated, "The stages of grief that family members go through are very similar to the stages of adjustment to death."[1] When Hughes was in the earlier stages of the disease, I did sometimes feel like a widow. But I do not feel like one now. Rather, I feel that I am in the process of coming full circle in my life, as if I have returned to the days before I knew Hughes, my earlier days of being a loner. But even though I had always enjoyed being a loner, with all my heart I still missed the Hughes I married.

As a caregiver I had to handle his body daily in giving him intimate care. Before AD, touching had given great pleasure, but now it was different. It had to be perfunctory and detached, strictly a matter of the business of keeping his body clean.

In adjusting to my new life, I had to review and reinforce what I believed about sexuality, and broaden and redefine my understanding of the meaning of intimacy.

A NEW INTIMACY

Before Hughes had AD I rarely thought of intimacy except as it related to sexuality. But the meaning of both sexuality and intimacy has evolved and broadened since I was a bride in the 1940s. For example, back then it was widely believed that after a certain age one could no longer perform sexually. But now studies indicate that older women and men can lead active sex lives well into their eighties or older.[2] In recent years many elderly people have freely spoken on television talk shows of their sexual successes.

I knew there was little in life more indicative of our humanness than our sexuality, and that we were sexual beings from birth to death. Sexuality was necessary for the propagation of the species, and we all came about because of it. Overall, I accepted that feelings of sexuality are normal, natural, and human at any age. I also knew that the sex drive has been characterized by some scientists as one of the strongest in humans. But when our four children became teenagers, I felt compelled as never before to make a greater distinction between our sexual desires and our basic needs.

Our children were teenagers at the height of the sexual revolution in the 1960s.[3] Change was rapid, the social pressures were great, and we had no guideposts or "how to" books. It was every parent for her- or himself. The demands of the time were driving us. I was desperate to help our children safely through this period. As a middle-aged parent counseling our teenagers on sex, I was challenged to examine and evaluate my own sexual maturation. I asked myself, had I matured beyond the adolescent fixation on sex? How much of myself (as an adult) was I seeing in our teenage children? Were my fears for them driven by my own sexual immaturity?

In searching for answers to these questions, I discovered that, indeed, my sexuality was a part of my codependency with Hughes. I also discovered that sex was just another form of energy, and although it was natural to desire it, we as humans had been given the ability to choose the ways we use our energy. This realization forms the core of the beliefs that I hold today on sexuality.

In the 1960s I had read the work of Swiss psychiatrist and psychologist Carl Jung.[4] He was a student of Sigmund Freud but broke with his teacher over the issue of sexuality. Freud believed that all our behavior was somehow related to sex; Jung declared that he did not believe his brain was an appendage of his genitals. In America I believe we have merged our wants and desires with our needs. It is my sense that in so doing, we have lost our way to personal restraint and personal accountability and have thus excused ourselves from self-control. Fusing of needs with wants also trivializes what is essential for every nation that hopes to endure: a strong sense of what is most valuable in life. This conscious process of reviewing and reaffirming my beliefs helped me to see sexuality from a much wider perspective, to define it not as relating almost exclusively to the act of sexual intercourse but much more broadly as including other kinds of physical touching.

Nevertheless, as Hughes lost more and more of his memory, I missed the intimacy more than anything else. We had shared intimacies in every detail of our lives together. One night I dreamed that Hughes and I had been separated for a long time; I did not understand why, but finally, I was going back to him. I was eager and smiling as I approached him, happily anticipating our getting back together again. I could hardly wait! But when I went in to see him, he acted strange. Suddenly a woman with wet hair, wearing a robe and carrying a steaming skillet of food, came out of the kitchen. Hughes had gotten another woman while I was gone! I could not believe it, and I felt an incredible, overwhelming loss. I did not cry; I could only moan and groan under the weight of so heavy a loss. The next morning when I awoke, I was so glad to see Hughes! I hugged him and greeted him with a deeper sense of appreciation than ever. I had never experienced such an incredible sense of bereavement in real life. Perhaps the dream was nature's way of helping me accommodate the tremendous loss I have felt since Hughes has had AD.

I decided to research the meaning of this intimacy I had lost. I read widely on the subject, and I discovered a whole new way of thinking and looking at it. I learned that in addition to sexual intimacy, there are several other types: emotional, social, intellectual, and recreational.[5]

In its broadest terms, intimacy was best defined for me in an article about Laurel Van Ham, a family practice counselor who defined intimacy as "knowing the internal reality of another person and letting that person know your internal reality, all in an atmosphere of unconditional acceptance." Van Ham asserted that "knowing yourself, intimately, is the foundation of intimacy with others." Culture, she said, "messes us up because we have this phrase that 'two people were intimate' and we mean sex. . . . If that's the only way of being intimate, there are other parts of life that aren't being tapped," because "aside from sexual closeness, intimacy can be spiritual, intellectual or aesthetic—like watching a sunset with a neighbor, enjoying a ballet with a co-worker, being part of a prayer circle, participating in an advocacy campaign, or playing racquetball regularly with friends."[6]

Van Ham went on to say, "It is a myth in our culture that we are going to find that one person with whom we can share everything—politically, playfully, intellectually, creatively, aesthetically." For most of our marriage I had felt it a betrayal of Hughes to share intimacies with others, but Van Ham suggested that people should "open themselves up to opportunities around them." I realized that was what I had to do. For example, I missed debating politics and current events with Hughes, but once I broadened my understanding of intimacy, I discovered that our son Eric was a natural partner in discussion and for sparring with me on any controversial subject. I saw him in a new light, and this gave our relationship new dimensions of respect and equity. Expanding my view of intimacy gave me a new life.

Hughes and I now share a new kind of intimacy, a nurturing unspoken kind that reaches out from the heart. My love for Hughes is stronger today than ever before. Other caregivers have expressed similar feelings.[7] For the first time in our marriage, I understand the meaning of unconditional love. As for sexuality, I have found several choices available to the spouse caregivers of a sexually active AD patient.

First, there is sexual intercourse. The well spouse may be potent for years beyond her or his partner's interest or ability to perform sexually, since it seems that the sex drive of the person with AD will gradually disappear.[8] Consequently, one must ask, what are my expectations of the patient? Are they the same as before AD? Is it realistic for me at this point in my life to expect one who is now demented to meet my needs? Am I taking unfair advantage of a person with AD? Confronting and dealing with these issues as they occur will help to reduce guilt and other negative feelings that can cause both partners emotional stress. Personal honesty at this time helps us to avoid future heartbreak.

Second, sexuality can be experienced and appreciated in its broadest sense: the physical closeness of hugging, kissing, stroking, caressing, snuggling, touching. Persons with AD continue to be human beings despite their mental deterioration and may thus have an ongoing need for this kind of physical intimacy. The caregiver might consider this form of sexual expression as the patient becomes impotent.

Third, there is the option of abstinence. When no sexual intercourse or sexual intimacy is possible or desired, the caregiver's energies are freed to explore new areas of personal growth, development, and creativity that heretofore might not have been plausible or practical.

REWARDS

The psychoanalyst Erik Erikson, writing about the different stages of life in his book *The Life Cycle Completed*, calls old age a time of wisdom or despair.[9] Most in-home caregivers are sixty-five or older. I see myself daily making choices between wisdom and despair. When we are young, generally, we are not learned and experienced enough to view events in our lives as parts, bits and pieces of a whole. That is why when we are young, we live and die by the daily events in our lives. But when we are old, we can view everything, including our present problems, from the perspective of a lifetime. For instance, I see these present travails as but one glitch in the span of our two lifetimes. "Weeping may endure for a night," the psalmist writes, "but joy cometh in the morning."[10] Suffering through to this perspective at any age makes wisdom possible, and out of this wisdom one is able to acknowledge and appreciate with deepest gratitude the rewards of caregiving.

These rewards are a study in the paradoxes and the mysteries of life whereby good comes out of bad.[11] The concept that good can come from bad, or that one is incomplete without the other, is central to many of the great philosophies and religions of the world. In traditional Chinese cosmology, for example, yang is the name of the "positive principle . . . in nature," which "combines and interacts with its opposite yin [negative principle] to produce all that comes into existence."[12] In Buddhism, it is believed that a "resolute faith can transform any suffering into benefit. This concept is known . . . as 'changing poison into medicine.'"[13] Christianity teaches that through belief in Jesus Christ, the son of God, all suffering can be transcended and turned into ultimate joy.[14]

The late Jacqueline Kennedy Onassis, former first lady of the United States, once said, "I have been through a lot, and I have suffered a great deal. But I have had lots of happy moments as well. . . . You cannot separate the good from the bad."[15]

The Gospel of St. Matthew quotes Jesus as saying, "Take my yoke upon you. . . . For my yoke is easy, and my burden is light."[16] Of course, it is against human nature to volunteer for yokes or to think of rewards and benefits in the midst of the harsh and relentless discipline required of the self in caregiving. That is why the rewards are so sweet when they do emerge out of the hardships. The rewards are gifts, as it were, that return to the giver. In other words, everything I do for Hughes I am in reality doing for myself. This is called the law of causality in Buddhism, and it teaches that for good or for evil, the effects of our actions invariably return to us. The teachings of Hinduism maintain that each person is the product of his or her past deeds. Christianity teaches that we reap what we sow.

I take care of Hughes in order to be able to face and live with myself. I am not a martyr; I do this not so much for Hughes as for myself. I do this to be true to myself and to my beliefs. Thus, the rewards are entirely personal and always accrue to the self. The rewards are ethereal, and they relate to humankind's search throughout human history "to know thyself," to conquer oneself, and to find meaning and purpose for one's life.

NEW INNER GROWTH AND PERSONAL DEVELOPMENT

Many years before Hughes had AD, the sisters told me that "there is a Hitler in all of our basements." I have seen mine many times over the years. But the sisters also said, "If you can see it, then you don't have to be it." In my moments of rage, anger, and rebellion, I have seen new depths of my human depravity; and I continue to confront it daily, since we are not made yet, not finished working on ourselves until we die. The sociologist and teacher Robert N. Bellah wrote in his book *Beyond Belief,* "I learned to see the darkness within, that we are all assassins in our hearts. If I am not a murderer it is because of the grace I have received through the love and support of others, not through the lack of murderous impulses within me. The only difference between me and the man on death row is that he somehow received less grace."[17] John Bradford, the sixteenth-century English Protestant martyr, is said to have commented upon seeing criminals led to their execution, "But for the grace of God there goes John Bradford."

As a caregiver, in my determination not to succumb to my depravity but instead to do a good job and also to survive whole, I continue to discover untapped wells of internal strengths and inner resources. Jesus said, "The Kingdom of God is within you."[18] So what do I do when Hughes does not understand how to get into the car on a freezing cold Nebraska day? I have to pray more often and dig deeper and deeper within at each new level of his deterioration. In so doing, I learn that there is still more patience and yet another answer to a problem. I learn to walk with him away from the car, leaving the door open, and then walk him back into the car. If that does not work, *something* works every time—mostly patience.

One's beliefs and faith have to become working, active instruments for surviving whole. Unlike the prayers of past years, words rushed through as a morning or evening ritual, prayers have become all-compelling as the only means I know for satisfactorily facing crisis after crisis with Hughes and successfully getting through each day. Now I understand a little better what

Brother Lawrence meant when he wrote that "it was a great delusion to think that the times of prayer ought to differ from other times. . . . Prayer was nothing else but the sense of the Presence of God."[19] Thus, one of the rewards has been a faith expanded to new levels of prayer, understanding and patience, perseverance and endurance, courage and creativity—and still I miss the mark. Yet an ever expanding faith enriches and fulfills one's life. I believe that the pain and discipline required to bring about the necessary changes in the caregiver create a new organism. Paul Tillich speaks of "the New Being, the New Creation." He writes, "The New Creation is healing creation because it creates reunion with oneself. And it creates reunion with . . . others."[20] It is this reunion with ourselves that makes us whole.

NEW SENSE OF SELF AND SELF-RESPECT

As a result of repeatedly confronting and resolving the daily difficulties involved with caregiving, plus the total responsibilities of managing a home, the caregiver receives a new awareness of her or his abilities and a new sense of identity. Accomplishing nontraditional tasks for women of my generation—cleaning and replacing furnace parts, trimming trees, tuck-pointing the house foundation—revealed a self I never knew existed. This awareness builds self-confidence about the future and what is possible. As the person in charge, I have also had to develop some degree of fearlessness. For example, early one morning, still half asleep after getting up in semidarkness, I was reaching for my washcloth when suddenly something hit my leg and fell to the floor, moving slowly as it spread its wide, dark wings in the half-light. I was so frightened I could not move momentarily, though I heard myself squeal. Who would have dreamed that a *second* bat would get into the house? Finally, I remembered to pray, and once again I secured Hughes's room, swished the bat to the basement, and called animal control. I decided that the meaning of the bats getting in was that I should never again be afraid of them. Such experiences have given new meaning to my determination never to feel defeated in any area of my life.

Taking care of Hughes has also increased my self-respect. I believe I should take care of him not out of duty but because it is the right thing for me to do. There is nothing in life more important than being able to live with oneself.

SENSE OF PURPOSE, SENSE OF BEING NEEDED

Since Hughes now has the cognition of a baby and needs help from the time he awakens until he goes to sleep at night, I never have to wake up wondering what there is today for me to do. Hughes needs to go to the bathroom. He needs a drink of water. He needs his face and hands washed. Someone needs me. This gives extra value and purpose to my life and enhances my desire to stay alive, to be active, and to keep healthy.[21]

HEIGHTENED SENSE OF PRIORITIES

A caregiver lives on the edge, never knowing from moment to moment or day to day what the person with AD might do or what the caregiver him- or herself might have to do. The result is a reorganization of priorities. For example, if I have gotten up several times in the night to clean and change Hughes, I am much less inclined the next day to get involved in pettiness or to be upset by daily trifles. In the past, a plumbing emergency or an appliance breakdown was a major calamity—but no more. When a machine breaks down, I know it is only something material, and that it can be fixed or replaced. The demands on my time and energies to administer to Hughes's basic human needs give me a keen ability to ferret out the important from the nonsense.

NEW INDEPENDENCE

It is paradoxical that it was Hughes's total dependence on me that gave me my independence. When I had to take over all the family responsibilities, make all the decisions, and work to supplement our income, I found my freedom. This new independence is an example of yin and yang, and also of "changing poison to medicine."

There were moments in Hughes's illness when I would gladly have welcomed the daily hassles and compromises necessary to keep a marriage honest and working for both partners. There were times when I prayed for his memory to return so that we could resume the life we had together. I wanted to shed all this responsibility and hide away once again in the security of his strong arms. Yet today, even if a miracle drug suddenly came on the market and restored his memory, I could never go back to living the way we did before AD. Those days are like a lost innocence, gone forever. I can not imagine voluntarily agreeing to be a dependent again.

I am thankful for every day that I am given to take care of Hughes, and each additional year gives me hope for the future. What I once felt to be a heavy burden is now routine. As humanity evolves, individually and collectively, I believe we can come closer to experiencing the inexplicable essence of life in all human beings, especially in loved ones who have contributed directly to our lives. Lest we forget, these are our brothers and sisters, our mothers and fathers, husbands and wives, grandmothers and grandfathers, sons and daughters—people whose task now is to live in the world of dementia.

Once in great despair I prayed, "Lord, how long will I have to continue to do everything for this man?" The answer came back, "Until you get it right."

I have not gotten it right yet, but most days I do it better. I believe it is in the grand design of life that taking care of an Alzheimer's patient should be as natural to us as breathing. The breath of life is so precious, so priceless. Now is the time to seize this moment of life and find it in our loved one.

Epilogue

It has been three years since I turned in the final manuscript for the hardcover edition of this book. It has been only six months since my sweet love, Hughes, died in my arms. Yet today, both of those life-altering events seem like blurred dreams from a life lived aeons ago. Perhaps that is the reward when one learns to live in the moment rather than in the future or the past.

After turning in the manuscript in late 1995, I plunged into learning how to give Hughes loving and competent care in the final stage of his life with AD. No one in the medical profession told me Hughes had entered the terminal stage, but I learned from Reisberg's Global Deterioration Scale (on page 14). In retrospect, I believe Hughes spent about two years in the last stage. I mark the beginning of his steady and final decline from a bad case of influenza in February 1996, despite his having had his yearly flu shot.

Before I learned about heel protectors, Hughes had developed several huge water blisters on his heels after spending only a few days in bed with the flu. The Veterans Administration nursing staff taught me how to clean and dress his wounds, and since Hughes continued to walk (with assistance), and maintained a hearty appetite until the last few months of his life, by late spring the sores had completely healed. But the illness had taken its toll, and by March 1996, after attending day care for eight years, he was discharged. His care now exceeded the day-care center's stated criteria. I told Hughes playfully that he had flunked day care.

However, I immediately enrolled Hughes in the only other adult day-care center in Lincoln at that time, Tendercare, which he attended for four months until the center closed. The new center was one mile from our home, and in the beginning, Hughes and I walked there and back. But he became increasingly confused about walking, sometimes plopping down suddenly, and in general dawdling like a small toddler, even though he remained a strong walker.

In May 1996, Hughes had the first of five grand mal seizures. Each seizure occurred while Hughes was toileting. His doctor prescribed Dilantin, but I was never sure if the medication helped. It made him drowsier, and if left unattended he would sleep in his chair the entire day. The seizures were difficult for both of us, but I learned to make those violent seconds tender, special moments for holding Hughes close to me. He usually slept for hours afterward, and I came to accept them as a necessary means of giving him some form of personal release. Throughout Hughes's long illness, I had practiced giving thanks for all things, and the seizures were no exception.

By the fall of 1996, I realized I was going to have to lift Hughes more and more, since he had long ago lost the cognition enabling him to get up on his own. I enrolled in a weight-lifting class at the local senior center and learned how to lift without hurting myself. I loved weight training! I could see and feel the new muscles in my arms. And though I was sixty-nine years old, this training gave me greater self-confidence for what I might have to face in the future. I also bought a lift chair that brought him up to a standing position. After Hughes fell down our front steps, skinning his knee, I had a Wheelovator (an outside elevator) installed at the front of our house. Neither Medicare nor our health insurance covered any part of either expense, even though both lifts enabled me to continue to take care of Hughes in our home.

Also in 1996, our nineteen-year-old granddaughter, Carrie, who lived in La Grande, Oregon, called to say, "I would like to come and stay with you and help you take care of Grandpa." I welcomed Carrie with open arms since Hughes was now at home twenty-four hours a day. But with paid sitters, along with Carrie, Eric, and Sherry (our family members in Lincoln), plus friends and some strangers who volunteered, I was able to continue to exercise, occasionally go out to dinner, and keep some out-of-town speaking engagements. I was still able to go on with my life.

Hughes's VA doctor ordered a hospital bed, mobile commode, wheelchair, and patient lift for transferring Hughes from his bed to the wheelchair. These were the major necessary assistive devices I needed in the final stage to help me as Hughes continued his relentless decline.

On Easter weekend, 1997, Carrie and I drove Hughes to Oklahoma City to see my sister, Claudine, one last time. At age seventy-seven, Claudine had heart disease and could not travel. I knew I would have to go to her, and Hughes's doctor saw no reason why I could not take Hughes on a nine-hour car trip to Oklahoma. The weather was perfect, and the drive was heavenly. When my sister saw Hughes in his deteriorated condition, she surmised that it had taken a herculean effort for us to come and visit her. I believe she understood for the first time the deep love that I felt for her. She died of a heart attack four months later.

Our family and friends gathered on Thanksgiving weekend, 1997, for our fiftieth wedding anniversary celebration. By now Hughes could no longer sit up on his own or smile. It was difficult for our children to see and accept that their father now had the abilities of a two- to three-month-old child. But overall, we had a good time.

Hughes stopped walking altogether in December. He also began to choke on his food at every meal, eating less and less. In January, he had another bout with the flu and developed another water blister on his heel. I began grinding his food and giving him food supplements. In February, Hughes's doctor told me he needed hospice care. The hospice workers who came to our home for the next five weeks were angels in disguise, especially our aide, Leachen. Every day Hughes ate less and less and slept more and more. He seemed to have no physical pain and appeared to be peaceful and at rest.

We got Hughes up and wheeled him to his lift chair each day except for the last week of his life. By now he would take little nourishment or water. The last time Leachen tried to feed him, he stated plainly, "Leave me alone."

I had never seen anyone die before, and I had no idea what to expect. But Hughes "told me." In the last two or three weeks of his life, he withdrew from me and into himself in a way that told me he was moving on to another world.

Two days before his death, I wanted desperately to get some recognition from him—anything, any sign that maybe he knew me and that maybe he knew how much I loved him. On an impulse, I asked him, "Honey, will you be my guardian angel?" And to my great surprise, with his eyes closed, he bowed his head once in the affirmative. I was alone and unbelieving. Again that night with Eric and Leachen present, I asked Hughes, "Did you really mean it when you said you would be my guardian angel?" This time he bobbed his head up and down several times vigorously! The next morning I asked him the same question a third time, and once again he nodded energetically. I believe it was then that I felt that after fifty years I could finally let him go.

He died quietly and magnificently in my arms on April 10, Good Friday. On April 13, our hospice aide's sister had a baby girl whom she gave up for adoption. Eric and Sherry brought the new babe home from the hospital and adopted her. They named her Lela.

Since Hughes's death, my life has changed, yet many things have stayed the same. One month later, I resumed my speaking schedule. Preparing for two major speeches in May helped me to get an early start on the transition to a new life. Contrary to popular belief, I do not feel a great sense of relief, because I had long ago stopped regarding Hughes's care as a burden. My days are filled with writing, reading, and speaking, and on special days I get to care for Baby Lela.

Also, through a miracle of serendipity, there is now a new friend in my life, a wonderful man who read this book and reached out to me to share his similar experience. There is a new spring in my step, a new joy in my heart, and all is right with the world.

Appendix

Outline for Primary Caregiver Training Course

I. Objective: To help beginning caregivers refocus and develop their own individual plan for a healthy survival and a proficiency in caregiving that will enable them to have some mental stability and also space and time for themselves.

II. Two suggested areas of training

A. Self-management (Objective: to assist caregivers in developing a plan that will permit them to go on with their lives)

    1. Coping strategies

    2. The discovery and development of hidden inner strengths

    3. Anger control and beyond

    4. The relationship of attitude and actions

    5. Sexuality and the patient

    6. Financial and legal counseling, with referral as needed

B. Management of the patient (Objective: To present solutions and alternatives, thus reducing caregivers' initial feelings of hopelessness, anxiety, and stress)

    1. Information about the disease and explanation of the patient's behavior

    2. Instruction in techniques for daily problem solving

        a. How to get the patient up (and out, if necessary) in the morning

        b. How to get the patient ready for bed

        c. How to give the patient a bath

    3. Tips on restructuring the home environment and the use of assistive devices

    4. Suggestions for communicating non-verbally with the patient

    5. Role playing to learn how to work with the patient

    6. Hearing experienced caregivers who speak realistically yet positively about their lives

III. Group therapy sessions as support (Objectives: To provide a support group that meets the individual needs of all different categories of caregivers; to provide training on a continuum; to provide guidance in moving from problems to solutions; to encourage personal growth as caregivers adapt to and establish a new life separate from the patient)

A. Follow-up on earlier training

B. Latest information about the disease

C. Open atmosphere for expressing one's feelings

D. Division into Subgroups as needed

    1. Beginning-stage caregivers

    2. Middle-stage caregivers

    3. Third-stage caregivers

    4. In-home caregivers

    5. Nursing home caregivers

    6. Long distance caregivers

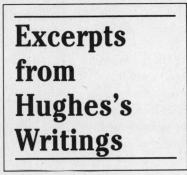

Excerpts from Hughes's Writings

An excerpt from a twelve-page epic Hughes wrote in 1943 describing his experiences in World War II.

THE ODYSSEY OF THE 855 ENGINEER AVIATION BATTALION

PART I

The Departure.......

> Early the morn of October twenty-eight
> The transport El'Kopiton steamed out the Golden Gate;
> Alone. Two-thousand men going overseas.
> The 855 Battalion, C. of E.

Life Aboard Ship.......

> The good ship plods a sou'west direction
> Midst calisthenics, rifle and hatch inspection.
> Ten o'clock, abandon ship drill
> Done to suit the Captain's will.

Fourteenth Day

> Three days off the Fiji Isles, our lookout
> Sights a British Bomber, we're all smiles.
> "Torpedo Junction" they call this spot
> Because Japanese Subs keep it hot.

PART II

Catastrophe. . . . . . .

> November eleventh, five forty in the morning
> I stand on deck stretching and yawning.
> As I watch the water I gasp for breath,
> For speeding our way comes sudden death.
> Torpedo!!! I cried, off the starboard bow!!!
> Too late, too late; our guns boom now.

Who Dares Command?. . . . . . .

> Men jumpin', oily water,
> Sharks approach from ev'ry quarter;
> Captain shouts, "Rafts!" We let 'em go
> Killing many who swim below.

PART III

Rescue (The First). . . . . . .

> The good ship Morriston comes our way
> And saves two hundred men today.
> Its Captain carries orders for a nonstop trip
> But loudly he cries, "Stop the ship!"
> Defies his orders and threat of court-martial,
> T'wixt orders and mercy to mercy he's partial.

Rescue (The Second)

> Just fore darkness falls o'er the sea
> A plane is heard by Brown and me.
> A giant seaplane takes forty men;
> "That's all this trip, be back again."

The Castaways

> Huddled close, chilled to the bone,
> Yet each man still feels all alone.
> "Mom once said she feels when I'm in trouble;
> Does telepathy traverse this 'big blue bubble'?
> I'd say 'all's well' if I could write;
> God grant she doesn't feel this night!"

Rafts drift far, in two long days,
Toss'd by furious ocean waves;
Roughest days we've seen so far;
Ironic, yes, but such is war.
Nite dark and eerie, faces drawn;
We pray, "Oh, God, please rush the dawn."

Joy.......

"Mast Ahoy! On yon horizon";
Wobbly legs on rafts a risin';
Oil fill'd eyes strain and peer;
"A U.S. Destroyer" (we shout and cheer).

Rescue (Final).......

Hauled aboard in hasty fashion,
Given food and coffee ration;
Sailin' roun' to pick up others;
Friend greets friend like long lost brothers.
Some in need of medic care;
Eyes blind beyond repair.

PART IV

Sojourn In Suva.......

Off to Fiji, rest in Suva.
(Heal quickly soldier, MacArthur needs ya'.)
Telegraph home: all is well
(just 'bout all you're 'lowed to tell).

New Caledonia.......

Ridin' at anchor, ships of all nations;
Linin' the shores, men of all stations;
Many races, creeds and faces
Gathered here from many places;
United in cause, tho' different in birth,
Preservin' democracy, fightin' for earth.

Reunion.......

We camp on a hillside o'er lookin' the sea;
'Bove windin' roads. "What's that I see?"

A truck convoy, hear the noise?
"Hey, Gang, fall out, here comes the boys!"
There's Parker, Skipper, and Chicago Red!
Why hell, we thought you guys wuz dead!
Strong men weep; a slap on the shoulder;
(Even the timid seem more bolder;)
We welcome many whom we used to hate.
Boy, oh, boy, reunion's great.

Roll Call. . . . . . .

"Fall in formation at regular places."
(We gaze forlorn at vacant spaces.)
Roll call shows there is much absence.
Names unanswered cause reminiscence.

PART V

Back To Sea. . . . . . .

"Pack up men, we sail tomorrow;
Forget your pain, cast out your sorrow;
Our Battalion motto is: Can Do.
Push on, we must, 'til war is through."

EPITAPH

Your names be remembered, you died not in vain:
Expendable you were, 'twas not Tojo's gain.
Without seeing a battle your lives were lost
But we shall win no matter the cost.
Some day we shall meet face to face
But first I must earn a right to that Place
And win your approval of my deeds here on earth
In defense of America, land of our birth.
I'll meet you some day and share leaven;
Wait for me there—the gates of heaven.

A children's story Hughes wrote in 1947.

CANDYLAND

Once upon a time there was great woe in Candyland. You see, for many centuries it had been the custom to hold a National Castor Oil Week, during which all of the people, young and old, were given a large dose of castor oil. Now this was very necessary because it had been learned that this was the only way to avoid having a tummy ache epidemic during the summer months in Candyland.

But now the people were complaining: "Castor oil," they said, "was harder to bear than a tummy ache." All through each winter and spring they slept uneasily, dreading the coming of June when they must take castor oil. This year there were mumblings, loud as thunder in the Chocolate Mountains. The people vowed that come June, they would revolt rather than take castor oil.

Thus was King Yum Yum greatly disturbed, for he was a good king and loved his people; and didn't the royal family detest castor oil too? So the king called in all of his scientists and told them, "Something must be done!!" And quicker than you can say "na koo," the scientists solved the castor oil problem. And here is the way they did it:

For a long time, they had been experimenting with vitamin pills and concentrated food tablets and had found them to be quite nourishing; so all they had to do was put on candy coatings and give them to the storekeepers.

This was done quicker than you can say "na koo," and joy reigned again in Candyland. There were no tummy aches and castor oil was banished from the land.

But lo and behold, new problems arose: first of all, there was widespread unemployment; for a dozen or so scientists could turn out enough pills and tablets for the millions of people, and the great candy factories were completely shut down. And too, the children became unruly. They had to be severely punished (for who cared about a threat of being sent to bed without his vitamin pills). Even the king was dissatisfied with the diet. At night after a heavy supper of five food tablets, he belched and burped but couldn't taste a thing, and his sweet tooth ached for candied yams with toasted marshmallows.

So the whole kingdom was agitated and there was an epidemic of sweet toothaches.

Now there came one day to Candyland a delegation of merchants from the Land of Milk and Cream. And they came to buy all of the sugar which was to be found in Candyland. Of course, there was a surplus of sugar now that candy was no longer manufactured, but King Yum Yum hesitated to sell. He was a wise king.

The foreign merchants were well received and a great feast was held in their honor. They were fed plenty of wineballs and became quite drunk and talkative. King Yum Yum began to question them and when he had learned all that he wanted to know, he summoned his chief engineer and gave him secret orders.

Quicker than you say "na koo," the candy factories were reconverted and the people were back at work.

The great cotton candy machines turned out giant cones of ice cream and sherbert with five scoops, each a different flavor; the pink lemonade fountains in the parks spurted malted milk and the flavors changed every day; the scientists worked night and day turning out new formulas for sundaes, cherry flips, and malted milks; tiny tots who had been extra special good were rewarded with popsicles instead of lollypops. And lo and behold, the country was swept by an epidemic of chubby cheeks and smiling faces.

And that is why in our country 'til this very day there is an ice cream store and soda fountain near every school, for our wise men have said it must be thus.

A letter Hughes wrote in 1961.

RACIAL DISCRIMINATION ON THE JOB

2600 North 12th Street
Kansas City 4, Kansas
August 16, 1961
Mr. James M. Quigley, Employment Policy Officer
Department of Health, Education and Welfare
Washington, D.C.

Dear Sir:

Your recent correspondence to my wife was a severe blow to my hopes that something would be done by the Bureau about its color problem. We trusting Negroes go on hoping that someone in authority will do something about the things we feel we shouldn't have to protest because these things are a matter of universal knowledge. We know that every step we wish to take, whether up, down or lateral requires someone's recommendation—and we know that any "protests" we make at any time is the kind of "talking back" that just isn't tolerated by the white boss who immediately brands us as "troublemakers" and so goes the "recommendation."

In desperation I am prepared to make the following accusations and am prepared to face those I accuse at my own expense.

1. I was told by Mr. Joseph S. Sewall, mgr., the Denver District Office, that I had no chance of promotion or of being rated eligible for promotion in his office because I am a Negro.

2. This same Joseph S. Sewall denied me the right to seek an advance of per diem for the required bureau training at Baltimore when I entered bureau employment in 1956.

3. This same Joseph S. Sewall also by withholding information, denied me the opportunity to request an advance of moving expense costs at the time I was granted promotion transfer to the Kansas City Payment Center.

The tragedy, sir, is that on occasions two and three I was not aware that I was being discriminated against. I call these situations discrimination in employment or promotion because at either time if I had lacked sufficient funds, I could not have qualified for that position. I do not believe bureau regulations required this undue hardship be placed on me or my family on either occasion. I could speak volumes about this hardship.

Your correspondence confuses me, what does constitute a complaint? Are you actually unaware that these conditions exist and must someone tell you that something is amiss before you can start house cleaning? My impression is that the President of the United States created a special committee which would take positive action to right existing evils and which would not act only after my people repeat anew complaints they have repeated over and over again for ninety-six years. I honestly like Joseph S. Sewall and preferred to believe that he only voiced the policies handed to him from higher up. However, if it will help my people I must sacrifice him as I have sacrificed myself.

In reply to your good wishes—I do not like Kansas City because it is bad for my health. Ten years ago I moved from this climate because it aggravated my war wounds. I made the move because it was impossible to further endure the mental anguish of working under the conditions as officially revealed to me in the Denver Office.

Very sincerely yours,

Hughes H. Shanks

An excerpt from an article Hughes wrote for Nebraska Report, *a publication of Nebraskans for Peace, January 1983.*

A LETTER TO MARTIN KING

(With apology to William Wordsworth's "London, 1802")

> Martin, you should be with us in this hour:
> Life has need of thee: for all creation
> Lives under threat of annihilation via radiation.
> Oh! rise up, return to us again;
> And give us the virtue to protest this shame.
> Thou hadst a voice whose sound was like the sea:
> Pure as the naked heavens, majestic, free,
> So didst thou travel on life's common way,
> In cheerful godliness; and yet thy heart
> The lowliest duties on itself did lay.

You never visited my town; but, oh, how you affected its people. My earliest recall is of your impact on my wife. It was Denver 1956 and her sorority was haggling over sending twenty-five dollars to your bus boycott fund. The debate on this issue followed a near unanimous vote to spend two hundred dollars for a cocktail party. Before the conclusion of that meeting, my child-like bride became a woman. She resigned and walked away in protest never to return. . . . You never visited our town, Martin. . . . But, oh, how you affected our town. Neismith, Swomley, Farnsworth, Hoyt, Connell are some of the many who crossed the Kaw [River] again and again to join the families picketing.

We came to Washington in August 1963, and I heard you, Martin; I heard you loud and clear; but I did not see you from where I stood while sharing your dream.

Martin, on the fifteenth anniversary of your April 4, 1967 address, Clergy and Laity Concerned republished that speech: "Beyond Vietnam: A Prophecy of the '80's." Reading it is like listening to you deliver it all over again. . . .

Martin, do you hear us?

A portion of the last formal talk Hughes gave, 26 May 1985.

SPEECH TO BLACK STUDENT ACTIVITY BOOSTER CLUB

Greetings to all students present whether you are graduating from high school or college or kindergarten or somewhere in between. You are probably glad you won't have to go to school for the next ten weeks.

My purpose here today is to pass on to you favors done by dedicated adults who helped me and other youth get started in the adult world of jobs and careers. . . . (They all voiced a similar creed that said: Favors should be passed on to those who need one; not returned to a benefactor who feels blessed that he had something to share.)

I graduated from high school in June 1936. Your grandparents most likely have told you that the graduates of 1985 face a job market today in which jobs are as scarce . . . as they were in the 1930's. . . . But for 1985 Black students there is a much broader area in which to seek a job or start a career than existed for Black students in the thirties. Thanks to our equal employment opportunity laws, theoretically, you are employable anywhere; but in actuality that may not be so due to the racial attitudes of some employers. The only way you can find out whether a business will hire you is that you apply for a job with that business. Let's call this Rule Number One for job hunting: you must apply for a job.

I have known so many Black job seekers who will not apply for a job at an establishment that has no Blacks already on their payroll. If you feel that way, you should ask yourself whether you are looking for a job or a friend. This comes under Rule Number Two: most people are supported by a job that pays a salary—friends don't pay salaries to friends.

A job interview is a chance given a job applicant to make a favorable impression using mainly his appearance to sell him- or herself. My Rule Number Three says the most favorable impression you can make is to enter and exit the interviewing place with an air and a bearing that says to all: "I belong here."

Equally important is Rule Number Four which warns: if asked what can you do, do not say, "I can do anything." Say: "I will try anything that needs doing." Be positive and state specifically what jobs you have held. Do not be ashamed to say, "Newsboy for X number of months or years," or "Mowed lawns for X number of customers for X number of summers," or "Shoveled snow for X number of customers for X number of winters." Rule

Number Four should also be followed when filling out a written application.

Speaking positively in this way permits the interviewer to recognize your ability to stick to a job and thus gauge your dependability, thus seeing you as worthwhile to train because your past record shows your stick-toitiveness.

Remember: Maybe you can do anything, but how do you prove this before you are permitted to demonstrate it? Following Rule Number Four may give you a head start in being hired ahead of the guys who say "everything."

In conclusion, I want to remind you, most likely you will always have to confront some racial prejudice. If you use it as a crutch or as an excuse, it will cripple you. Or, just as you can learn to walk through a door with a bearing that says you belong there, you can also learn to walk with a bearing that says: I am a man or I am a woman. I am a person. I am not a color.

Reflections from Others in Hughes's Family

Nena St. Louis is a critically acclaimed playwright, performer, and visual artist.

"People will not open doors for you," Daddy once told me. I seethed with anger every time I remembered him saying that. If the truth be told, I seethed with anger every other day—because that's how often I remembered. It must have been a good lesson if I still remember it, even though I often tell other people that my father was too hard on me. My father and I are a lot alike. In fact, we're so much alike, we both have diseases of the brain. Last year I was diagnosed as a schizo-affective. Everyone who knows me was surprised because I am an overachiever with a very full life. In the last few months I've realized that if my father hadn't been so hard on me, if he hadn't told me in advance that people wouldn't open doors for me, I wouldn't have such a full life. I'm happy that my mother believed hard enough that a person with a brain disease has the right to have as full a life as he's capable of having.

Cedric M. Shanks is manager of the Union Wallowa County Community Corrections Program in La Grande, Oregon.

The first and most important decision I had to make was accepting my father's condition: that this college-educated man was no longer capable of being my father—because of Alzheimer's disease. That was not easy, and it hurt (and occasionally it still hurts). However, I knew I had to accept his present condition or it would tear me up. How can words contain the apprehension that preceded confronting his deterioration, or the painful grief for the father I once knew who will never return although he still breathes, smiles, and frowns before me? Then there is the sadness that a man of such intelligence and resourcefulness now has the mental capacity of a toddler.

As I look into those large moist brown eyes of a man who was incredibly wise—thinking before he acted and teaching me to do the same—I long to give him the big bear hugs he always resisted but doubtless secretly enjoyed. This man, my father, continues to teach me about life and about myself. How can I separate how I feel about him "now that he has Alzheimer's disease"? I cannot.

When I was thirteen I started playing golf. I remember my father caddying for me. Although he had never (to my knowledge) played the game, because he was a "thinker" he had a good grasp of the basic concepts. Through observation and thought, he sensed how certain shots should be played to get the best results. I of course thought I knew more as the one who actually played the game. However, by applying his notions, my game improved dramatically. And now, I too think, and I have learned the value of his input beyond nine holes of golf and into my life as a whole.

How do I feel about my father? I feel that there is still much for me to learn from him—and I love him for that (amongst a hundred other reasons).

Shela Omell Richards is a mother, performance artist, and director of operations for a nonprofit organization in New York City.

When I was fifteen I played a joke on my father to have some good adolescent fun. I entered the house with a friend and announced, "Guess what Daddy, I'm pregnant." Pretending to pay attention, he glanced from behind his newspaper smiling and said, "That's nice." Many years later I related this story to my husband, Jim, when my father couldn't remember his name during their first meeting. I just laughed it off saying, "He's always been absentminded." The fact was, that day my father had continually called me "Carolyn," his younger sister's name. He had also apologized over and over to my brother Ron saying, "I'm sorry I can't remember your name." Somehow, I just regarded it all as "Daddy being Daddy." When he asked for the tenth and fifteenth time during dinner, "Where are we? Why are we here?" I giggled and patted his knee to quell his impatience.

Over the next couple of years, I lived a protected and self-centered life a thousand miles away. I didn't worry too much about the accounts of my father's bizarre behaviors in my mother's letters. My father was still "my hero": a brilliant intellectual who exemplified the words courage, integrity, and compassion. When he and my mother came to visit following the birth of my second child, I was expecting both of them to take care of me. In retrospect it seems that my own sanity must have been temporarily suspended. My father was clearly inexplicably paranoid and appeared to be hiding things from my mother. He was confused about the function of ordinary objects and again, consistently called me Carolyn. He was unclear about who Jim was, and several times a day asked him what he thought of "that new baby" as if Jim was not the father. I refused to become alarmed, convinced that he was just "going through something"—something that could be fixed.

When I received an "official" letter from a physician stating that my father was believed to have AD, I was determined that I would pray him back to normality. Buoyed by false hope, padded by denial and illogical reasoning, I was determined to surprise everyone by not becoming emotional over the facts—which I had yet to make a part of my reality.

A few years later my husband, three children, and I visited my parents. The visit was just short of disastrous. I looked in my father's face and realized he had no idea who I was. He battled with my sons over toys, put my eight-month-old baby down to walk, and required personal assistance in much the same way my children did. Coming home had always meant a chance to refuel on my parents' nurturing. This time I found my father out of touch and my mother's energies absorbed in his care. The child in me was screaming, "This is not the way it's supposed to be!" I felt a sense of loss for both my mother and father. I drew my arms tighter around my own children—angry, confused, overwhelmed—grieving. I was happy when the visit ended—relieved that we lived far away. On the more positive side, confronting this reality head-on caused me to replace my prayer for my father's "cure" with a prayer for his and my mother's happiness, no matter what. Without realizing it, I was beginning to make the facts of my father's illness a part of my reality, and a new relationship with him and my mother could now begin to take shape.

Two years ago I went to Nebraska alone to take care of my father. It was a tremendous privilege to brush his hair and bathe him. I experienced great joy when he lovingly cooed to a musical doll I had brought for him. It was a wonderful feeling to share my Buddhist prayers with him when I put him to bed.

My father is now beyond the point of calling me by any name. Accepting that he has AD has opened the way to a beautiful relationship that has given me a greater understanding of the value of human life. When I look into his eyes, I see a man whose life has exemplified courage, integrity, dignity, and wisdom; a man who cared deeply for others and is deeply loved; a happy man, whose life continues to bring joy to others: my father.

Eric Hughes Shanks is a writer.

My mother and I talk about the misguided attitude people often show when they tell us how "sorry" they are about my father having AD. We lament for them when they tell us how "terrible" it is that he "isn't himself" anymore. He still gives me a lot. I guess the things that they think we are missing in him are all the things that made him who he was. Past tense. He didn't stop giving and we haven't stopped taking what he gives.

There are lots of things that make him who he is. Things that make me who I am. Things I couldn't give myself. Simple things. I've probably spent more time thinking about things he's given me, and is still giving, than what I might have lost. There are two things that stick out in my mind. I have a name only he could've given me, and when I wear a hat, I wear it his way.

My father used to slightly tilt his hat. His own characteristic tilt (now mine) was as flashy as he ever got. I used to love the way he did that. It was all he needed, too. No frills. He still tilts it the same way now. Each morning that I take him to adult day care, I tilt his hat for him a second time. It has become a kind of joke with some of the staff and the more lucid clients who laugh when I do it. They think I'm poking fun at him. They don't understand that he will always correct it with the precise tilt I remember as a boy. And that gives me joy.

My father's first name is also my middle name. I was always glad it was given to me even before it meant anything to me. That name gave me my freedom. It gives me strength far beyond what I could've gained on my own. The Hughes family name is the only part of our family tree that I've looked up. It gave me concrete proof that my people are more than just the offspring of freed slaves. I knew he never acted differently, but I didn't know why. Learning the reason made me feel stronger. His people's people owned land and went to college. So now, when I drop my first name and use my middle one, I'm screaming loud and high, "Hey, we ain't just a bunch of expatriated Africans! We're landed and educated, too!" That's a kind of freedom he gives me.

Christopher M. Shanks, grandson of Hughes, is fourteen years old.

I came to Lincoln about a year ago not knowing what to expect. I had heard about Alzheimer's from my grandma, but only the basic details. What I didn't anticipate was a grown man that couldn't take care of himself. He didn't know how to do anything himself. It was like watching a seventy-five-year-old baby. It didn't have any emotional effect on me, because as far back as I can remember he's had Alzheimer's. So I've just grown to accept it. When he sits down on the couch with his head up, he looks like one of the most intelligent people. He still has most characteristics he's probably had all of his life: calm, sweet, and caring. I like to help take care of my grandpa. It's fun to spend time with him, probably 'cause I love him so much.

Notes

INTRODUCTION

1. Shannon Talkington-Boyer and Douglas K. Snyder, "Assessing Impact on Family Caregivers to Alzheimer's Disease Patients," *American Journal of Family Therapy* 22 (spring 1994): 57–66. According to Karen K. Noel, executive director of the Alzheimer's Association, Lincoln, Greater Nebraska Chapter, at present there are approximately forty thousand AD patients in the state of Nebraska; by the year 2000 the number is expected to rise to seventy-seven thousand.

2. The national office of the Alzheimer's Disease and Related Disorders Association is located at 919 North Michigan Ave., Chicago IL 60611–1676. An 800 number, or the address of a local chapter, can be found in many phone books or by calling directory service.

3. *National Directory of Educational Programs in Gerontology and Geriatrics,* 6th ed. (Washington DC: Association for Gerontology in Higher Education, 1994).

4. Quoted in Joseph P. Lash, *Eleanor and Franklin* (New York: Norton, 1971).

CHAPTER I   HOW ALZHEIMER'S STARTED IN HUGHES

1. See his letter to James M. Quigley in the appendix.

2. Gary D. Miner et al., eds., *Caring for Alzheimer's Patients* (New York: Plenum Press, 1989).

CHAPTER 2   THE THREE STAGES OF THE DISEASE

1. See Barry Reisberg, M.D., et al., "The Global Deterioration Scale for Assessment of Primary Degenerative Dementia," *American Journal of Psychiatry* 139 (September 1982): 1136–39; Manfred Bergener and Barry Reisberg, eds., *Diagnosis and Treatment of Senile Dementia* (Berlin: Springer-Verlag, 1989).

2. See Steven H. Zarit, Nancy K. Orr, and Judy M. Zarit, *The Hidden Victims of Alzheimer's Disease: Families under Stress* (New York: New York University Press, 1985).

3. Zarit, Orr, and Zarit, *Hidden Victims.*

4. See Miner et al., *Caring for Alzheimer's Patients;* Ronald C. Hamdy et al., *Alzheimer's Disease: A Handbook for Caregivers* (St. Louis MO: C. V. Mosby, 1990).

5. Miner et al., *Caring for Alzheimer's Patients.*

6. Howard Gruetzner, *Alzheimer's: A Caregiver's Guide and Sourcebook* (New York: Wiley, 1992).

7. Gruetzner, *Alzheimer's.*

8. Hamdy et al., *Alzheimer's Disease.*

9. Nancy L. Mace and Peter V. Rabins, *Thirty-six-Hour Day* (Baltimore MD: Johns Hopkins University Press, 1991).

10. Mace and Rabins, *Thirty-six-Hour Day.*

11. Reisberg et al., "Global Deterioration Scale," 1136–39.

12. Mace and Rabins, *Thirty-six-Hour Day.*

13. Mace and Rabins, *Thirty-six-Hour Day.*

14. Zarit, Orr, and Zarit, *Hidden Victims.*

15. Mace and Rabins, *Thirty-six-Hour Day;* Mary E. Exum et al., "Sundown Syndrome: Is It Reflected in the Use of PRN Medications for Nursing Home Residents?" *Gerontologist* 33, no. 6 (1993): 756–61.

16. Bergener and Reisberg, *Diagnosis and Treatment,* 91.

17. Mace and Rabins, *Thirty-six-Hour Day,* 110; Reisberg, "Global Deterioration Scale," 1138.

18. "Place" used here as in Matthew 24:15.

CHAPTER 3   THE HUMANITY OF THE ALZHEIMER'S PATIENT

1. Daniel Callahan, in Robert H. Binstock, Stephen G. Post, and Peter J. Whitehouse, eds., *Dementia and Aging: Ethics, Values, and Policy Choices* (Baltimore MD: Johns Hopkins University Press, 1992), 141. I disagree with Callahan's support of age-based medical-care rationing.

2. See Gruetzner, *Alzheimer's.*

3. Albert Deutsch, *The Mentally Ill in America* (New York: Columbia University Press, 1967).

4. Lincoln Regional Center, "Rebuilding Lives . . . Together" (brochure), Nebraska Department of Public Institutions, Lincoln, Nebraska.

5. Robert Bogdan and Steven J. Taylor, "Relationships with Severely Disabled People: The Social Construction of Humanness," *Social Problems* 36 (April 1989): 135–48.

6. *Hamlet* 2.2.

7. Quoted from Lela K. Shanks, "Alzheimer's Disease: Creative Survival" (videotape, 1989).

8. *King Lear* 1.4.

9. See Binstock, Post, and Whitehouse, *Dementia and Aging.*

10. U.S. Bureau of the Census, *Statistical Abstract of the United States, 1993,* prepared by the Economics and Statistics Administration, Bureau of the Census (Washington DC, 1993).

11. In Binstock, Post, and Whitehouse, *Dementia and Aging,* 13.

12. American Federation of Government Employees, Social Security Local No. 1336, 601 East 12th Street, Kansas City MO.

CHAPTER 4   EARNING TO LIVE IN THE WORLD OF DEMENTIA

1. See Lars Backman, ed., *Memory Functioning in Dementia* (Amsterdam NY: North-Holland, 1992).

2. Katherine Bick, Luigi Amaducci, and Giancarlo Pepeu, eds., *The Early Story of Alzheimer's Disease* (New York: Raven Press, 1987), 2.

3. Miner et al., *Caring for Alzheimer's Patients.*

4. See Gruetzner, *Alzheimer's.*

5. Kathleen D. Mayers, "Calming the Agitated Demented Patient: Use of Self-Soothing Techniques," *American Journal of Alzheimer's Care and Related Disorders and Research,* July/August 1994, pp. 2–5.

6. Miner et al., *Caring for Alzheimer's Patients.*

CHAPTER 5   THE ALZHEIMER'S PATIENT AND CLEANLINESS

1. Robert N. Butler, M.D., *Why Survive? Being Old in America* (New York: Harper and Row, 1975).

2. Quoted in Edward L. Schneider, M.D., and Jack M. Gurainik, M.D., "The Aging of America: Impact on Health Care Costs," *Journal of American Medicine* 263, (2 May 1990): 2340.

3. Margaret Walker, *For My People* (New Haven CT: Yale University Press, 1942), 14.

4. Butler, *Why Survive?*

5. See Steven Long, *Death without Dignity* (Austin: Texas Monthly Press, 1987).

6. Hamdy et al., *Alzheimer's Disease.*

7. Hamdy et al., *Alzheimer's Disease.*

8. Naomi Feil, "The Validation Method," *Alzheimer's Caregiver* 7 (December 1993): 1–2.

CHAPTER 6   THE IMPORTANCE OF ESTABLISHING PROCEDURES

1. Jitka M. Zgola, *Doing Things: A Guide to Programming Activities for Persons with Alzheimer's Disease and Related Disorders* (Baltimore MD: Johns Hopkins University Press, 1987).

2. Zarit, Orr, and Zarit, *Hidden Victims.*

3. Zarit, Orr, and Zarit, *Hidden Victims.*

4. Deepak Chopra, M.D., *Ageless Body, Timeless Mind: The Quantum Alternative to Growing Old* (New York: Harmony Books, 1993).

5. Dorothy H. Coons, ed., *Specialized Dementia Care Units* (Baltimore MD: Johns Hopkins University Press, 1991).

6. Zarit, Orr, and Zarit, *Hidden Victims.*

7. Bergener and Reisberg, *Diagnosis and Treatment.*

CHAPTER 7   DEALING WITH PROBLEM BEHAVIOR

1. Zarit, Orr, and Zarit, *Hidden Victims.*

2. Viktor E. Frankl, *Man's Search for Meaning* (Boston: Beacon Press, 1992), 148.

3. Norman Cousins, *Head First: The Biology of Hope* (New York: Dutton, 1989).

4. Quoted in Shanks, "Alzheimer's Disease."

5. Gruetzner, *Alzheimer's.*

6. Ralph Waldo Emerson, "Compensation," from *Essays: First Series,* in *The Complete Works of Ralph Waldo Emerson* (New York: A.M.S. Press, 1968), 2:125.

7. See Ralph E. Lapp, "The Einstein Letter That Started It All," *New York Times Magazine,* 2 August 1964.

8. Jiska Cohen-Mansfield, Perla Werner, and Marcia S. Marx, "The Impact of Infection on Agitation: Three Case Studies in the Nursing Home," *Ameri-

can Journal of Alzheimer's Care and Related Disorders and Research, July/August 1993, pp. 30–34.

9. Senate Committee on Labor and Human Resources, Subcommittee on Aging, "Nursing Home Residents' Rights: Has the Administration Set a Land Mine for the Landmark OBRA 1987 Nursing Home Reform Law?" 102d Cong., 1st sess., staff report, 13 June 1991.

10. Miner et al., *Caring for Alzheimer's Patients;* Mace and Rabins, *The Thirty-six-Hour Day.*

CHAPTER 8   TWENTY COPING STRATEGIES

1. Richard Schulz, Paul Visintainer, and Gail M. Williamson, "Psychiatric and Physical Morbidity Effects of Caregiving," *Journal of Gerontology: Psychological Sciences* 45, no. 5 (1990): 181–91.

2. Zarit, Orr, and Zarit, *Hidden Victims.*

3. Melody Beattie, *Codependent No More* (New York: Harper & Row, 1987).

4. Paul Tillich, *The Shaking of the Foundations* (New York: Scribner, 1948), 50–51.

5. Clyde Reid, *Celebrate the Temporary* (New York: Harper & Row, 1972), 43.

6. *Wellness Review* (Public Relations Department of Lincoln General Hospital), summer 1993.

7. Quoted in Earl Ubell, "The Deadly Emotions," *Parade,* 11 February 1990, pp. 4–6.

8. Alexis Carrel, *Prayer* (Ridgefield CT: Morehouse, 1948).

9. A. J. Russell, *God at Eventide* (New York: Dodd, Mead, 1965), 148.

10. Nebraska Department of Social Services, "Treatment of Resources and Income When Your Spouse Needs Assistance," IM-PAM-45 Rev. 11/92 (99250).

11. Nebraska Department of Social Services, "Waiver Services for Aged Persons," MS-PAM-6 2/90 (99106).

12. Nebraska Department on Aging, "Long-Term Care Ombudsman Program: Providing a Helping Hand through Advocacy and Mediation on Behalf of Residents of Long-Term Care Facilities" (brochure).

13. *The Journal of Katherine Mansfield,* ed. J. Middleton Murry (New York: Knopf, 1927), 167.

14. Jacqueline M. Stolley, "When Your Patient Has Alzheimer's Disease," *American Journal of Nursing,* August 1994: 34–40.

15. Norman Cousins, *Anatomy of an Illness* (New York: Norton, 1979).

16. Cousins, *Head First,* 132.

17. See Butler, *Why Survive?*

18. Maurice Nicoll, *Psychological Commentaries on the Teaching of G. I. Gurdjieff and P. D. Ouspensky* (London: Robinson & Watkins, 1973).

19. *The Way of a Pilgrim and The Pilgrim Continues His Way*, trans. R. M. French (New York: Seabury Press, 1965).

20. Quoted in Mrs. Chas. E. Cowman, comp., *Springs in the Valley* (Grand Rapids MI: Zondervan, 1969), 89.

21. Fritz Kunkel, M.D., *Creation Continues* (New York: Scribner, 1952).

22. Lawrence Kushner, *Honey from the Rock* (Woodstock VT: Jewish Lights, 1992), 89.

23. Chopra, *Ageless Body, Timeless Mind*.

CHAPTER 9   FINDING RELIEF FROM TWENTY-FOUR-HOUR CAREGIVING

1. M. Powell Lawton, Elaine M. Brody, and Avalie R. Saperstein, *Respite for Caregivers of Alzheimer Patients: Research and Practice* (New York: Springer, 1991).

2. "Adult Day Care Centers Vital, Many More Needed," *Journal of American Medicine* 269 (12 May 1993).

3. Count of Residents in Nursing Homes in Nation, Total and Those with Dementia, Nursing Facilities and Skilled Nursing Facilities (U.S. Department of Health and Human Services).

4. Publication of the National Eldercare Institute on Long Term Care, National Association of State Units on Aging, 1225 I Street NW, Suite 725, Washington DC 20005.

CHAPTER 10   THE FUTURE FOR ALZHEIMER'S PATIENTS AND CAREGIVERS

1. Lawton, Brody, and Saperstein, *Respite for Caregivers*, 2.

2. Alzheimer's Disease and Related Disorders Association fact sheet, *Alzheimer's Disease Statistics*, August 1991, ED 230Z.

3. *American Journal of Public Health*, August 1994.

4. *Advances in Alzheimer's Research* 3 (fall 1993): 1.

5. Eric Pfeiffer, in "Alzheimer's Disease Research: Latest Findings and Application," National Eldercare Institute on Long-Term Care and Alzheimer's Disease teleconference, 26 April 1994.

6. Theresa Tighe, "Drugs, Treatment Ease Alzheimer's Grip," *St. Louis Post Dispatch*, 5 December 1993, sec. D, pp. 1, 10; Stuart L. Nightingale, M.D., "From

the Food and Drug Administration, Tactrine Hydrochloride," *Journal of the American Medical Association* 267 (15 January 1992): 339.

7. Robin Marantz Henig, "Alzheimer's," *New York Times Magazine,* 24 April 1994, pp. 72–76; K. A. Fackelmann, "Anti-Inflammatories: New Hope for Alzheimer's?" *Science News* 145 (19 February 1994): 116.

8. *Alzheimer's Association Newsletter* 14 (fall 1994): 7; A. Nitta et al., "Effects of Oral Administration of a Stimulator for Nerve Growth Factor Synthesis in Basal Forebrain-Lesioned Rats," *European Journal of Pharmacology* (Amsterdam) 250 (30 November 1993): 23–30 (MEDLINE, National Library of Medicine, AN: 94206041); A. Seiger et al., "Intracranial Infusion of Purified Nerve Growth Factor to an Alzheimer Patient: The First Attempt of a Possible Future Treatment Strategy," *Behavioural Brain Research* (Amsterdam) 57 (30 November 1993): 255–61 (MEDLINE, National Library of Medicine, AN: 94161882).

9. Allen D. Roses in *Alzheimer's Association Newsletter* 13 (winter 1993); B. Wuethrich, "Higher Risk of Alzheimer's Linked to Gene," *Science News* 144 (14 August 1993): 108; P. St. George-Hyslop et al., "Alzheimer's Disease and Possible Gene Interaction," *Science* 263 (28 January 1994): 537; T. Brousseau, et al., "Confirmation of the e4 Allele of the Apolipoprotein E Gene as a Risk Factor for Late-Onset Alzheimer's Disease," *Neurology* 44 (February 1994): 342–44.

10. Genica Pharmaceuticals Corporation, *The ApoE GenoType Report: Questions and Answers about Diagnostic Risk-Factor Assessment for Alzheimer's Disease,* April 1994, 2.5M (pamphlet).

11. *Discover,* December 1993, p. 30.

12. *Alzheimer's Association Newsletter* 13 (winter 1993): 4–5.

13. Colleen L. Johnson and Leslie A. Grant, *The Nursing Home in American Society* (Baltimore MD: Johns Hopkins University Press, 1985).

14. Chopra, *Ageless Body, Timeless Mind;* Cousins, *Head First.*

15. Coons, *Specialized Dementia Care Units.*

16. Zarit, Orr, and Zarit, *Hidden Victims;* Senate Special Committee on Aging, "Reducing the Use of Chemical Restraints in Nursing Homes," 102d Cong., 1st sess., 22 July 1991.

17. Coons, *Specialized Dementia Care Units.*

18. Johnson and Grant, *Nursing Home;* Carter C. Williams, "Long-Term Care and the Human Spirit," *Generations,* fall 1990, pp. 25–28.

19. Moyra J. D. Jones, "Gentlecare: A Prosthetic System of Dementia Care to Change the Experience of Dementing Illness," lecture presented at the Ninth Conference on Alzheimer's Disease International, September 1993, Toronto (audiotape, Audio Archives International).

20. *Friends of the Eden Alternative* 1, nos. 1–2 (1993); see also *USA Today,* May 17, 1993, pp. 1D–2D.

21. Mary Buzzell, "Personhood and Hope: Two Concepts in the Care of Those Affected by Alzheimer's Disease," lecture presented at the Ninth Conference on Alzheimer's Disease International, September 1993, Toronto (audiotape, Audio Archives International).

22. S. D. Gilster, "Innovative Specialized Care for persons with Alzheimer's Disease: An International Perspective," lecture presented at the Ninth Conference on Alzheimer's Disease International, September 1993, Toronto (audiotape, Audio Archives International).

23. Chari Weber, "Innovative Specialized Care for Persons with Alzheimer's Disease: An International Perspective," lecture presented at the Ninth Conference on Alzheimer's Disease International, September 1993, Toronto (audiotape, Audio Archives International).

24. Coons, *Specialized Dementia Care Units.*

25. Ivy Winchester, "The Prototype Caregiving Program of the Future: A Touch of Class . . . a Caring Touch," lecture presented at the Ninth Conference on Alzheimer's Disease International, September 1993, Toronto (audiotape, Audio Archives International); Coons, *Specialized Dementia Care Units.*

26. Paul E. Larrat et al., "Development of Alzheimer's Disease Special Care Units on a Statewide Level," *American Journal of Alzheimer's Care and Related Disorders and Research,* March/April 1994, pp. 22–26. Eighteen percent of nursing homes in Nebraska have special-care units, according to Barbara McCabe, preliminary report presented to the Governor's Task Force on Alzheimer's Disease and Related Disorders, 20 October, 1994, Lincoln.

27. Coons, *Specialized Dementia Care Units.*

28. Gilster, "Innovative Specialized Care"; Jones, "Gentlecare."

29. K. L. Rocks, "Innovative Specialized Care for Persons with Alzheimer's Disease: An International Perspective," lecture presented at the Ninth Conference on Alzheimer's Disease International, September 1993, Toronto (audiotape, Audio Archives International).

30. Stolley, "When Your Patient Has Alzheimer's Disease."

31. Dianne Hurren, "Enhancing the Quality of Life at Home: Assistive Technology Devices and Quality of Life of Persons with AD," lecture presented at the Ninth Conference on Alzheimer's Disease International, September 1993, Toronto (audiotape, Audio Archives International).

32. Lynn B. Gerald, "Paid Family Caregiving: A Review of Progress and Policies," *Journal of Aging and Social Policy* 5 (1993): 73–89.

33. Publication of the National Eldercare Institute on Long Term Care, National Association of State Units on Aging, 1225 I Street NW, Suite 725, Washington DC 20005.

34. *Employment Guide* (Washington DC: Bureau of National Affairs, 1994).

35. Gerald, "Paid Family Caregiving."

36. Neena L. Chappell, "Implications of Shifting Health Care Policy for Caregiving in Canada," *Journal of Aging and Social Policy* 5 (1993): 39–55.

37. Joy Glenner and Lorie Van Tilburg, "Regenerations," *American Journal of Alzheimer's Care and Related Disorders and Research,* May/June 1994, pp. 2–6.

38. Letha A. Chadiha et al., "Targeting the Black Church and Clergy for Disseminating Knowledge about Alzheimer's Disease and Caregivers' Support Services," *American Journal of Alzheimer's Care and Related Disorders and Research,* May/June 1994, pp. 17–20.

39. *National Public Policy Program 1995,* Alzheimer's Association, Chicago (Edward F. Truschke, President; Stephen McConnell, Senior Vice-President for Public Policy).

40. Council on Scientific Affairs, "Physicians and Family Caregivers: A Model for Partnership," *Journal of the American Medical Association* 269 (10 March 1993): 1282–84.

41. Hubert Humphrey, Remarks at the dedication of the Hubert H. Humphrey Building, 1 November, 1977, *Congressional Record* 123 (4 November 1977): 37287.

CHAPTER 11   THE NEW LIFE OF THE CAREGIVER AND ITS REWARDS

1. Gruetzner, *Alzheimer's.*

2. Osborn Segerberg, *Living to Be 100: Twelve Hundred Who Did and How They Did It* (New York: Scribner, 1982).

3. Susan Sprecher and Kathleen McKinney, *Sexuality* (Newbury Park CA.: Sage, 1993).

4. *Carl G. Jung: Collected Works,* ed. Herbert Read, Michael Fordham, and Gerhard Adler; trans. R. F. C. Hull (Princeton NJ: Princeton University Press, 1953).

5. Sprecher and McKinney, *Sexuality.*

6. Quoted in Patty Beutler, "Sharing Intimate Moments," *Lincoln (Nebraska) Star,* 23 March 1992, p. 9.

7. Phyllis Braudy Harris, "The Misunderstood Caregiver? A Qualitative Study of the Male Caregiver of Alzheimer's Disease Victims," *Gerontologist* 33, no. 4 (1993): 551–56.

8. *A Guide to Living with Alzheimer's Disease: Caring for the Caregiver* (Morris Plains NJ: Parke-Davis division of Warner-Lambert, 1994).

9. Erik H. Erikson, *The Life Cycle Completed* (New York: Norton, 1982).

10. Psalms 30:5.

11. Jean Wood, "One Caregiver's Story—Grabbing the Gauntlet," *Alzheimer's Caregiver,* August 1993, p. 2.

12. *Webster's Third New International Dictionary,* 3d ed., s.v. "yang."

13. *Seikyo Times* (Santa Monica CA), no. 320 (March 1988): SGI-USA Publishers.

14. Tillich, *Shaking of the Foundations.*

15. Quoted in "Jackie Dies Peacefully at Home," *Lincoln (Nebraska) Journal,* 20 May 1994.

16. Matthew 11:29–30.

17. Robert N. Bellah, *Beyond Belief: Essays on Religion in a Post-Traditional World* (New York: Harper & Row, 1970), xvi.

18. Luke 17:21.

19. Brother Lawrence, *The Practice of the Presence of God,* trans. from the French (Old Tappan NJ: Revell, 1980), 24.

20. Paul Tillich, *The New Being* (New York: Scribner, 1955), 23.

21. Harris, "Misunderstood Caregiver?"

Index

FOR THE BEST IN PAPERBACKS, LOOK FOR THE

In every corner of the world, on every subject under the sun, Penguin represents quality and variety—the very best in publishing today.

For complete information about books available from Penguin—including Puffins, Penguin Classics, and Arkana—and how to order them, write to us at the appropriate address below. Please note that for copyright reasons the selection of books varies from country to country.

In the United Kingdom: Please write to *Dept. JC, Penguin Books Ltd, FREEPOST, West Drayton, Middlesex UB7 0BR.*

If you have any difficulty in obtaining a title, please send your order with the correct money, plus ten percent for postage and packaging, to *P.O. Box No. 11, West Drayton, Middlesex UB7 0BR*

In the United States: Please write to *Consumer Sales, Penguin USA, P.O. Box 999, Dept. 17109, Bergenfield, New Jersey 07621-0120.* VISA and MasterCard holders call 1-800-253-6476 to order all Penguin titles

In Canada: Please write to *Penguin Books Canada Ltd, 10 Alcorn Avenue, Suite 300, Toronto, Ontario M4V 3B2*

In Australia: Please write to *Penguin Books Australia Ltd, P.O. Box 257, Ringwood, Victoria 3134*

In New Zealand: Please write to *Penguin Books (NZ) Ltd, Private Bag 102902, North Shore Mail Centre, Auckland 10*

In India: Please write to *Penguin Books India Pvt Ltd, 706 Eros Apartments, 56 Nehru Place, New Delhi 110 019*

In the Netherlands: Please write to *Penguin Books Netherlands bv, Postbus 3507, NL-1001 AH Amsterdam*

In Germany: Please write to *Penguin Books Deutschland GmbH, Metzlerstrasse 26, 60594 Frankfurt am Main*

In Spain: Please write to *Penguin Books S. A., Bravo Murillo 19, 1° B, 28015 Madrid*

In Italy: Please write to *Penguin Italia s.r.l., Via Felice Casati 20, I-20124 Milano*

In France: Please write to *Penguin France S. A., 17 rue Lejeune, F–31000 Toulouse*

In Japan: Please write to *Penguin Books Japan, Ishikiribashi Building, 2–5–4, Suido, Bunkyo-ku, Tokyo 112*

In Greece: Please write to *Penguin Hellas Ltd, Dimocritou 3, GR–106 71 Athens*

In South Africa: Please write to *Longman Penguin Southern Africa (Pty) Ltd, Private Bag X08, Bertsham 2013*